UN-SIT
YOUR LIFE!

THE REFLEX "DIET" SOLUTION

Change your sitting habits
Empower your life

BARBARA & KEVIN KUNZ

To our friends Michael Kinneavy, Jill Schneider, Sandy Gooch,
Harry Lederman, Bob Hawley and Jean Hawley, and our parents
Margaret Kurcaba and Kaiser Kunz with thanks for your support

Published by RTS Publishing, New Mexico, USA
© 2015 Kevin and Barbara Kunz. All rights reserved.
ISBN 978-1515193616

Produced by **Bookworx**
Editor Jo Godfrey Wood
Designer Peggy Sadler
Proofreader Beth Hamer

DISCLAIMER
Every effort has been made to see that the information contained in the book is
complete and accurate. The ideas, procedures, and suggestions contained in this book
are not intended as medical advice. If you have a medical problem you should consult a
healthcare provider. Neither the publisher nor the authors accept any responsibility for
any personal injury or other damage or loss arising from the use or misuse of the
information and advice in the book.

Contents

About the authors

We are reflexologists, researchers, and authors of 19 books published in 21 languages. We have enjoyed a life-long study of the reflex actions influencing the body and health, prompted as pressure is applied in a systematic and targeted approach to the feet and hands: reflexology.

It was a newspaper article that drew our interest to sitting too much. We saw the resulting problems as happening when not enough pressure is applied to the feet as one sits rather than standing and/or walking. Researching the idea was fascinating, but we also un-sat our own lives. For Kevin the results were especially dramatic, with a weight loss of 40 pounds. For both of us, we've shaped up and become more energetic.

OUR MISSION

Our goal is to draw attention to the perils of sitting and the solution of un-sitting to help people become participants in their own wellbeing. To further this goal we created a system we hope both explains and encourages un-sitting. We present the reflex, automatic unconscious responses to what one does, as an explanation for why sitting has the impact it does on the body. The concept of "diet" draws attention to "dosing": how much and how often one needs to un-sit to create a desired result. With a "menu" of techniques we hope to illustrate the variety of ways one can un-sit one's life. Our goal is to create a guide to un-sitting, how breaking the habit of sitting can change your life and make you a participant in your own wellbeing.

About the reflex "diet"

In our mission to get us all out of our chairs and moving about more we have pulled together our own plan – or "diet". This includes:
→ Re-setting your metabolism for the modern age
→ Enhanced walking
→ Active sitting
→ Sitting less
→ Moving more
→ Systems to improve reflexes

We have drawn on the research of others to give the reader a fully rounded view of the subject.

IMPORTANT WORDS

We've used our own language to explain our solution to help us all change our sitting habits and to become more mobile in order to improve our health. You'll find the following terms used throughout the book in a slightly different way from their usual sense:

"Diet" The habits of sitting and moving about for the right amounts of time to achieve a healthy "inner you".

"Nutrition" Sitting, standing, walking, and movement (as "nutrients") to better use your reflexes to regulate the mechanisms that run your body, prompted by sitting smart and moving more to provide "nourishment".

"Dose" How much and how often one sits or moves about to achieve a result.

Part one

THE REFLEX "DIET" THEORY

1 Introduction to the reflex "diet"

Are you feeding your reflexes the right "diet" – the day-to-day sitting, standing, and walking experiences it needs to keep you healthy?

Before you answer that question, consider: does your body behave the way you want it to? Have you had problems keeping your weight in check? Is your blood pressure or cholesterol under control? Does sitting at work all day literally give you a pain in the neck or your lower back?

Our bodies and metabolisms are designed to stand and move about most of the time – not sit for most of the time.

It could be that your body and its reflexes are out of sync with the life they're meant to be living. We evolved over millions of years to do one thing: to move around. Our bodies and metabolisms are designed to stand and move about most of the time – not sit for most of the time. Muscles, joints, and ligaments are intended to hold us upright in a standing position – not a sitting one.

Our culture has created a chair-dwelling lifestyle, and we find ourselves sitting most of the time, whether at work, at home, at school, or when traveling from place to place. There is a fundamental mismatch between what our bodies are built to do and what they actually spend their time doing.

Our bodies were once accustomed to hunting and gathering food as a way of life and they had evolved and adapted to moving around much of the time as needed for such

WE ARE OUR ANCESTORS

We are our ancestors, inheriting our physical and mental selves, with wellbeing compromised by the experience of sitting for much of the time. The results are physical and mental conditions brought about by a lifestyle unsuited to our body's design.

a lifestyle. Since the move away from this lifestyle and into villages is a relatively recent occurrence for humans, it is seen that our "modern (urban) society" is inherently stressful. The constant walking about as well as the multi-sensory experiences in the outdoors, the sounds, sights, smells, and clean air are not so readily available to provide reflex "nourishment".

When we sit too much, move too little, and carry out the same sedentary activities over and over again, the reflex actions involved in moving us about don't get the workout for which they were designed. Metabolic, and other, processes are not practiced adequately, or enough, to maintain the operation of the human body as intended.

The result is disarray in how our body works, its metabolism, musculoskeletal system, circulation, and brain function. What follows is a cascade of events. Increased are risks for adverse lifestyle conditions such as stroke, heart disease, diabetes, obesity, and Alzheimer's. Decreased is longevity.

Coordinating the moving "you" with the inner "you" is under way continually, happening all the time as reflexes get to work in the background.

How do you make your body behave the way you want it to? It's important to realize that we are now chair-dwellers inhabiting cave-dwelling bodies, originally used to a far more active and challenging lifestyle. You then need to harness the reflexes used during sitting, standing, and walking to create an optimal metabolic imprint on your body in our present-day world of chair-living. The reflex "diet" can work with the way the body is designed to work, to help you build a better, longer life.

Harnessing your reflexes

"Reflex". The word conjures up thoughts of Pavlov and his experiments on the reflex reactions of dogs. A reflex is an automatic, unconscious response prompted by a stimulus. The reflex most of us are familiar with is the tap on the knee, causing the lower leg to fly up: the knee-jerk reflex. But there's a whole complex world of reflexes and reflex activities at work for us day and night, 24/7.

Actions such as sitting down and standing up, taking a step and breaking into a run all happen as automatic reflexes unconsciously direct the necessary body parts to do our bidding. Reflex activities of the inner "you" respond as well, adjusting our metabolisms to what we're doing. Standing and walking use up more energy than sitting, and running takes up still more. Coordinating the moving "you" and the inner "you" is under way continually, happening all the time as reflexes get to work in the background.

Ancient ancestors were biologically pre-programed to move for a critical period of time each day and we have inherited this. Lifetimes spent hunting and gathering food to survive pre-programmed our muscles and metabolisms, setting them to engage the inner "you" and our metabolism in the activities of standing and walking. There is no substitute, no amount of exercise, that can match the biological imperative of giving enough of a workout to this automatic, unconscious reflex system built to stand and walk rather than sit.

Have a seat – but be aware that your body is counting the minutes.

The reflex effect

Have a seat – but be aware that your body is counting the minutes, creating the reflex activity you've requested. Feed your reflexes the right stuff, the sitting, standing, walking, and movement "nutrients" in the right amounts, and you create a healthy "diet".

A positive reflex effect happens as we do what our bodies are designed to do: move about for the right amount of time. A negative reflex effect happens when we're inactive for too long, sitting and engaging in less activity than is needed to keep the inner "you" engaged and working.

Carry out enough positive reflex activities and the inner "you" receives a workout appropriate to staying well and fit. Sitting about for too long creates negative reflex activity, and the inner workings literally shut down, leading to disarray and, over time, chronic degeneration of the body.

Tapping into the reflex effect

Our reflex "diet" system provides exercise to the mechanisms that keep us moving. These are the mechanisms that are under-exercised as we sit for prolonged periods of time. The reflex "diet" provides information about how much and how often you move about to create a healthy inner "you".

Tapping into the reflex effect is all about time and timing, which we call the "dose".

Tapping into the reflex effect is all about time and timing, which we call the "dose", helping the reflexes do the job for which they were designed by interrupting sitting on a timely basis as well as being up and about more. Just as research has discovered how much sitting time impacts health negatively, research has revealed also how much interruption and moving about has a positive influence on wellbeing.

UN-SIT YOUR LIFE

No matter what kind of a day you're having, today could be the best day of your body's life. When you un-sit your life, shaping the activities of sitting, standing, walking, and moving to the best benefit, you'll know that you're building a better-functioning body as well as improving your overall health.

CASE STUDY: RE-SETTING THE REFLEXES

Kevin and researcher Dr. Avi Patel implemented some of the ideas to be explained in this book. Kevin "re-set" his reflexes by getting rid of his office desk chair and creating a standing desk. He used a standing station for his iPad for the evenings. He also used nubby reflexology mats underfoot. Dr. Patel added more steps to her day: parking further away from her office, walking at lunchtime, visiting colleagues in their offices instead of emailing. Each lost 40 pounds in weight. Kevin's weight loss has continued and he's now lost eight inches from his waistline. Kevin and Dr. Patel found the right amount of sitting, standing, walking, and moving activities for their bodies. They found the tipping point more closely matching their lifestyles to their cave-dwelling metabolisms and they harnessed their reflexes to shape the bodies they wanted.

The goal of tapping into the reflex effect is to help you better use your reflexes to regulate the mechanisms that run your body. The reflex effect is controllable. It's something you can do to prompt your body to behave in the way you want it to. Read on to explore how you can tap into the reflex effect, your body's natural balancing act.

Our reflex "diet" helps shape your current lifestyle to match your paleolithic-designed reflexes. Sitting, standing, and walking are tools to automatically and unconsciously feed your body the "nutrients" it needs for optimal upkeep.

The reflex "diet" provides "nourishment" for the mechanisms that keep us moving.

It's free. The only ingredients needed are you and your decision to commit your time to saving yourself from the risks of a chair-living lifestyle.

How does the reflex "diet" work?

Our reflex "diet" can teach you how to exercise the mechanisms that keep you moving. These are the mechanisms that are under-exercised as we sit for prolonged periods of time. The reflex "diet" tells you how much and how often you need to move about to create a healthy inner "you".

As you "feed" your reflexes the right stuff, you won't be randomly sitting, standing, walking, or moving about. You'll be working intentionally to achieve a natural balance between positive reflex activities (standing, walking, and moving) and negative reflex activity (sitting) to achieve your goal.

THE NEW "NUTRITION"

In a food diet, nutrition is extracted from what you eat. Food is the delivery method for the vitamins, proteins, minerals, and carbohydrates that are then processed by the body and provide nutrition to it. You have to consider carefully how much and what sort of food you eat to create a healthy intake of nutrition.

In the reflex "diet", "nutrition" comes from what you do. Sitting, standing, and walking are the delivery methods for the actions of core postural muscles and the foot's pressure sensors that are then processed by the body to provide "nutrition". You have to consider how often, how much, and what sort of activity you need to undertake in order to remain healthy.

Just as nutrition in food impacts the whole body, so too does the "nutrition" of sitting, standing, and walking. It is referred to as "tone". It is the state of readiness of the inner "you" to appropriately meet the demands of the day. You've probably heard of one state of readiness, "fight or flight". Well, rest and relaxation describe its counterpart. For the inner cave-dweller, balancing the two extremes involves sitting, standing, walking, and moving in appropriate "doses".

IF YOU DON'T LIKE IT, CHANGE IT!

Your body is under your control, so if you don't like it, change it! Don't like your metabolism? Change it! Your blood pressure too high? Lower it. Pounds don't seem to come off? Worried about your risk for Alzheimer's? Cancer? Stroke? Diabetes? You can lower your risk for each of these conditions.

You are what you do

Rocking provides more "nourishment" than sitting still.

You are what you spend your time doing. When you move about enough, you receive a workout enabling the cave-dwelling inner "you" to stay well and fit. Sit and remain inactive for too long and your inner workings literally shut down, leading to disarray and, over time, a less healthy body, with an increased risk for certain damaging lifestyle conditions. This happens because a footstep does more than move us about. A footstep happens as core postural muscles of the body contract and relax. Pressure sensors on the feet play a critical role, feeding important information about staying upright into postural muscles. The activity of core muscles and pressure sensors creates reflex actions, prompting metabolism into action.

You need to think about how much and how often you sit, stand, walk, and move about in order to prompt reflex actions that will "nourish" the inner "you". You also need to look at the level of activity involved in sitting, standing, walking, and moving about. For example, rocking in a rocking chair provides more "nourishment" than sitting still in an ordinary chair. Doing something while standing, such as washing dishes or playing with a pet, has more impact than not doing something. But take heart! You can overcome the problem of living in a chair-dwelling world whilst inhabiting a cave-dwelling body.

What can the reflex effect do for you?

Tapping into the reflex effect can put you in control of your health and wellbeing. Rather than rolling the dice where your

METABOLIC DYSFUNCTION

Metabolic dysfunction is one of the mechanisms thought to be at work linking prolonged sitting and increased risk of endometrial, ovarian, and prostate cancer. Some 30% of colon cancer and 21% of breast cancers may be due to physical inactivity. Those who worked in a sedentary job for ten or more years increased their risk for colon cancer by 44%.

health is concerned, realize that you're the boss, in charge, as you accentuate positive reflex activities and decrease the negative ones. You are manager of your own body. You decide where to put your resources to get to where you want to be.

There is an air of predictability about what happens as we move or not. Being up and about creates positive experiences for your reflexes and for you. Your health will thrive. Standing and walking are tools available to re-set our metabolisms, our musculoskeletal system, and other body mechanisms, and they are available for free, any time. Just stand up and walk! A window of opportunity opens to create dialogue with your inner self.

You can alter your metabolism – when you stand and move. If you don't stand and move enough, the fat circulating in your blood goes into storage. The more you sit, the bigger your waistline will become. The more you sit, the greater your increase in risk for obesity. Every two uninterrupted hours of television-watching in the evening increases the risk for obesity – by 23%.

Potentially, fat not used by the muscles for movement continues to float around in the bloodstream. The danger is that the fat becomes embedded in your blood vessels, risking the start of health problems such as stroke and heart attack. Every two hours of television-viewing increases the risk of cardiovascular disease by 15%, according to an analysis of four studies from the US, Europe, and Australia with a total of 34,253 participants conducted by Dr. Frank Hu of Harvard and Danish researcher Anders Grontved.

When you stand and move, you change your metabolism of sugar and insulin. Not standing and moving enough means that the sugar is not needed, so the insulin pumped into cells to activate it continues to circulate in the blood. Your body produces more, leading to a cycle. Each two hours of television-viewing increases the risk of diabetes for women by 14%. Six hours of uninterrupted sitting per day doubles the risk for diabetes. Each two-hour per day increment in sitting at work is associated with a 7% increase in diabetes.

You can alter your metabolism – when you stand and move.

As you move, your circulation is encouraged, with more good things happening: more blood is pumped to your brain and heart, helping them to work better and move more of the hormones that produce those feel-good moods through your body. Your vestibular apparatus, responsible for sensing balance and indicating body position, gets a workout as well. Benefitting also are blood pressure and heart beat, as the brain responds to standing or walking.

Your musculoskeletal system receives the breaks it needs, relieving the prolonged and deforming stretch of ligaments and muscles that occurs when seated. Strengthened by the demands of being upright as well are the bones, thus providing help with osteoporosis prevention. Veins embedded in the muscles of your legs propel more blood to the heart and brain as legs move, helping overcome potential insufficiencies in circulation from the extremities.

The reflex connection

A newspaper article began our exploration of what was to become our reflex "diet". The article was about Dr. Patel's study and she reported that women who sat for more than six hours a day during their time off had a 33% higher risk of early death from cardiovascular disease than women who sat for three hours. The figure was 18% for men. We realized that these people weren't getting enough pressure to their feet, since they were sitting so much rather than standing or walking.

Linking pressure and feet to health consequences was familiar territory to us. We are reflexology practitioners, authors, and researchers by career and we first realized the value of pressure to the feet when we worked with paralyzed individuals in 1980. What we saw, then, was that reflexology technique applied to a particular part of a paralyzed foot prompted movement of the opposite hand or foot. Literature research led us to understanding why this would be. We had tapped into deep pressure sensors in the bottoms of the feet, stimulating a part of the body's walking mechanism. In addition, technique application prompted growling of the stomach, sweating, or overall body shivering, responses of the paralyzed individuals' internal organs. As we found out, internal organs work together with pressure sensors in the feet to help manage the body's energy expenditure, its metabolism. As noted earlier, pressure sensors communicate whether one is sitting or standing or walking, each requiring a different level of energy expenditure.

What we saw was a reflex effect, automatic, unconscious responses of the body's tone as pressure was applied to the feet.

We realized what we saw was a reflex effect, automatic, unconscious responses of the body's tone as pressure was applied to the feet. The value of pressure to the feet was its

SIT WITH A PURPOSE, MOVE WITH A PLAN

With our reflex "diet", you'll sit with a purpose, the purpose of minimizing impact on your metabolism and the inner "you" when you sit. You'll move with a plan, a plan to maximize impact on your metabolism and the inner "you" while standing, walking, moving about, and engaging in purposeful activities.

DRAMATIC RESULTS

In our research we applied the reflex effect ideas to our own lives. We sat less, moved more, and utilized reflexology mats, walking barefoot on varied surfaces. The results for Kevin were dramatic. One day his trousers no longer fitted him. We then realized that he was losing weight – and that his un-sitting campaign was responsible, since neither his diet nor exercise had changed. He would go on to lose 40 pounds in weight and six inches from his waist in eight months, with a total of eight inches over time. And his weight and waist loss continued as his metabolism changed.

By this time, our study of prolonged sitting had found both an explanation for what happens as well as a goal. The goal was to create a system to combat the problem of not moving enough. The result is the reflex "diet", a "menu" of techniques and a "recipe" for "dosing" – how much and how often to apply to them.

ability to contribute to balancing basic states of readiness, fight or flight, and rest and relax.

The reflex effect explained the impact of reflexology technique application: shaping health and responses from the inner self, impacting lifestyle conditions, relaxation, and walking abilities.

"Dosing" and the reflex effect at work

"Dosing" was important: the systematic application of pressure to the feet over time produced the best results. It was these same ideas that we were to apply when we became aware of the problems of sitting too much. When we were writing an article and looking for an example of reflexes at work, we remembered Dr. Patel's article. Soon we couldn't get away from prolonged sitting – the idea, that is. Article after article, study after study – we became fascinated with what happens when we sit too much. It was the reflex effect at work. Utilizing not only pressure

SAVE YOUR LIFE WITH THE REFLEX "DIET"

We're trying to entice you to follow the reflex "diet" because we want to help you to better your life. Even if your life does not seem to be particularly "in danger", its quality can improve today, tomorrow, and from now on.

sensors of the feet but also postural muscles of the body had potential to impact the inner "you", on cognitive abilities, walking capabilities, and the basic human operating system.

Matching you to your lifestyle

The goal of the reflex "diet" is to more evenly match the cave-dweller inner "you" with your chair-dweller lifestyle. You'll make better functions of the inner "you" and lessen risk for lifestyle conditions by interacting with the basic building blocks of walking, the postural muscles of the body, and the pressure sensors of the feet.

The goal of the reflex "diet" is to more evenly match the cave-dweller inner "you" with your chair-dweller lifestyle.

So how do you "feed" your reflexes the right stuff, giving them enough of a workout to keep your metabolism and other systems working the best they can? How much sitting and how much standing, walking, or moving about creates the optimal impact on your metabolic and other reflexes? What can you do to optimize your sitting, standing, and walking time? Research provides the answers. Read on!

The reflex "diet": the right "dose"

We have spent many months sifting through studies to find the "nutritional" value of reflex techniques. From this we have created a system of "dosing", how much time spent in which activities will create for you the reflex "diet" to achieve your goals. As you work with the reflex "diet", you'll discover, in Part Two, which reflex techniques work best for you.

The basic idea is that you need to stand, walk, and move for two hours more a day than you do currently. Take a break from sitting preferably every 20 minutes for two minutes, but definitely at least once an hour for at least five minutes. We call this the "recipe for success". This will let you re-set your metabolism and musculoskeletal system as well as expend more calories. Time spent taking breaks counts towards the two hours, a five-minute break each hour adds up to an hour a day. This is the simplest way we can explain the "diet". If you stop reading here and follow this "dosing" formula, you will impact your life profoundly. This is the essence of what you need to do to change your life. Stick to it. Before you know it, you'll have an entirely different body.

Take a break from sitting preferably every 20 minutes for two minutes, but definitely at least once an hour for at least five minutes.

Timing provides you with the right "doses" of moving about to keep you healthy, target a health concern, and live longer. As you shape the amount of time you sit, stand, and move, you shape the body you want, behaving the way you want.

WHAT RESEARCH SHOWS

Why the reflex "diet" is going to work for you is backed by research, which shows that un-sitting your life most closely meets your body's overall needs, improving metabolic indicators and cognitive abilities, as well as maintaining weight and meeting musculoskeletal needs. The main research studies are highlighted throughout the book in special boxes.

Patterns for lowering risk for specific lifestyle conditions have also been established and are discussed in Chapter 10. Included are: cognitive abilities and decline/dementia/Alzheimer's, cancer preventive, diabetes prevention, cardiovascular disease, longevity, musculoskeletal concerns, weight, and more.

Studies have revealed how much sitting is associated with abnormalities created in metabolism, longevity, diabetes, cardiovascular disease, cognitive decline, and more. Research has found how much up-and-about time lessens risk for these lifestyle conditions.

Why sit two hours less a day?

What happens when people sit for two hours less a day, substituting sitting time for moving time? The answer is simple: they don't gain weight. Those who sit for an hour or two less a day than others have "better indicators" of metabolism, showing a lessened risk for lifestyle conditions such as diabetes and heart disease. We know this because of studies that assessed what

RESEARCH ON SITTING LESS

Dr. Genevieve Healy, of Australia, conducted a study whereby 4,757 participants wore accelerometers measuring activity during their waking hours for seven days. She found that those who sat for an hour to two less a day had better metabolic indicators for fats and sugars than those who sat the most. Those who took the most breaks had waistline measurements that were smaller by 1.6 inches.

Dr. Healy compared results for the 25% who sat the most with the 25% who sat the least. Her overall finding: "in theory, population-wide reductions in sedentary time of between one to two hours a day could have a substantial impact on the prevention of cardiovascular disease." Measured were: waistline, HDL ("good") cholesterol, and triglycerides as well as insulin resistance, a precursor to diabetes, and C-reactive protein, a marker for inflammation and indicator for cardiovascular risk. The goal was to link sitting time with "various indicators of risk for heart disease, metabolic diseases such as diabetes, and inflammatory processes".

MAXIMISING RESULTS

Not all sitting, standing, or walking is the same. Sit in a recliner and your metabolism receives less of a workout than if you sit up. Walk in place while standing and your postural muscles are more at work, creating more benefit. Do something as you walk about, such as playing with a pet – you'll expend more calories.

happens when people wear devices to measure what they do around the clock, in one case, or during waking hours in another.

It's in the way you move

Some people are mobile two hours more a day than others, engaging more in activities as simple as picking up a piece of paper. These are the people who keep their weight in balance.

It's the thousands of contractions of postural muscles as we move throughout the day that make a difference to our health and wellbeing.

Every move you make and every step you take has an impact on weight, metabolism, and more. Researchers state it's the thousands of contractions of postural muscles as we move throughout the day that make a difference to our health and wellbeing.

Reflex effects over time

Being mobile two hours more a day; taking two-minute breaks. It sounds simple enough and it is. But there's one more aspect of timing to think about. How long do I need to do this for? This is what your metabolic and other reflexes need every day. Think "recommended daily reflex allowance" – your new lifestyle.

Your life includes recommendations to keep you healthy and well. Think about the minimum daily requirement of vitamins and minerals you need to stay healthy and avoid nutritional deficiencies, which has been established by the Institute of Medicine. Look at any bottle of vitamins and you'll see the "% daily value" for each tablet or pill. Standards have been set for

RESEARCH ON MOVING MORE

The research of Dr. James Levine of the Mayo Clinic showed that individuals who were mobile two hours more a day maintained their weight and expended more energy than they required to stay alive. In the process of revving up their metabolisms, they staved off negative lifestyle conditions. His participants wore full-body motion-detecting suits for two months. They were asked not to exercise. He discovered the heavier among the participants stood and walked two and a half hours less a day (six and a half hours' total moving time) than their lean counterparts (nine hours a day total moving time).

Study participants ate only mandated food served at the laboratory, consuming a diet of 1,000 calories more than necessary to maintain body weight. At the end of the two-month study, some of the participants had gained weight (almost two pounds) while others had not (0.16 pounds). Those who gained weight engaged in fewer simple activities such as bending over to pick up something. Those who did not gain weight compensated for the extra calories taken in, moving about more, expending more energy. What did they do? "Their bodies simply responded naturally by making more little movements than they had before the overfeeding began, like taking the stairs, trotting down the hall to the office water cooler, bustling about with chores at home or simply fidgeting."

moderate-intensity physical activity of 30 minutes for five days a week to maintain general health and fitness.

We have created a basic reflex "diet" to meet the body's needs and give your reflexes the workout they need every day. Un-sit your life every day and you'll be fit for the rest of your life.

RESEARCH ON BIOLOGIC COMPONENT TO SITTING

Among conclusions from the study there is a "biologic" component to prolonged sitting. Some individuals just naturally move more and some just naturally sit more. A colleague on Dr. Levine's team, Colleen Novak, found an answer. Her research with rate led to the conclusion "… the brains of people with a tendency towards obesity don't respond to signals from their muscles or brains that tell them to move. And the more they sit, the fewer signals there are."

Intrigued by the idea that little movements throughout the day matter, Dr. Levine coined the term NEAT (NonExercise Activity Thermogenesis, or daily activities other than exercise). The idea that small movements throughout the day make a difference that can be developed as a solution to sitting too much caught on. Isn't it time you became a mover?

The reflex "diet" in action

Sit for two hours less each day; take a break from sitting every 20 minutes; do it every day. It sounds simple and it is. But there are ways to get more benefit from your efforts, ways to target your health interest, ways to motivate yourself. And that's where the reflex "diet" comes in.

Sitting too much uniquely contributes to many lifestyle conditions. Un-sitting your lifestyle allows you to take action in response to a health interest. For example, among the reflex techniques you'll read about, ten help lower blood pressure. Did you know that a sustained reduction in diastolic blood pressure can reduce risk for stroke by up to 56% or heart attack by up to 37%?

Need some motivation to get up and get moving? There are ways to quantify your efforts so you can know that what you're doing is proving beneficial.

Reflex techniques

You automatically and unconsciously feed your reflexes as you sit, stand, and move through the day. But as you have seen, the activities of the chair-dwelling lifestyle create problems for the inner cave-dweller.

Reflex techniques add focus and purpose to your day. You'll be "feeding" your reflexes the right stuff as you consciously plan the time and timing of your sitting, standing, walking, and moving about. Then there are the possibilities of enhancing, getting more from your sitting or up-and-about experiences. Once you create a plan and make it a habit, you'll have a lifestyle that becomes second nature to you.

Here are the basic techniques. They are described more fully in Part Two, with the all-important information about how much time creates what kind of results that form the reflex "diet".

Sitting smart

You'll be sitting smart by considering the chair in which you sit and what you do as you sit. How much sitting has what kind of impact is discussed in Chapter 5.

You'll be sitting smart by considering the chair in which you sit and what you do as you sit.

Did you know that the recliner is viewed as the "high heel of chairs"? This is because sitting in a reclining position is more impactful on the metabolism than sitting upright. If the recliner is a negative reflex generator, the rocking chair is a positive reflex producer. Did you know that using a rocking chair eats up twice the calories as when you are sitting still and is viewed by some as a therapeutic device, aiding recuperation as well as improving balance and walking mechanisms, mood and emotions, in addition to reducing pain?

Then there are the benefits of doing something as you sit. Reading, knitting, applying self-reflexology techniques or other forms of what's called "fidgeting" engage and benefit both your physical and mental selves. Then there are golf balls, spiky balls, or foot rollers that can be rolled across the foot or hand. If you have difficulties with being mobile, standing and walking, you'll want to consider the sitting smart techniques.

Taking breaks

Interrupting prolonged bouts of sitting is a technique in itself. As you will read on page 26, taking breaks in sitting does all sorts of good things: re-sets the metabolism, eats up calories, normalizes blood pressure and blood sugar, takes the stress off the musculoskeletal system as well as feeds more blood to the heart and more blood and nutrients to the brain. A five-minute break every hour is crucial. A two-minute break every 20 minutes is preferable. Wait until you hear the good things that result from frequent breaks. Did we mention a smaller waistline?

Move with a purpose

Think of nourishing the inner "you" with reflex actions resulting from thousands of contractions of your postural muscles and communications from pressure sensations to your feet at work as you sit less and move throughout the day more.

Take more steps

Every 1,000 steps taken or half hour spent on house-cleaning, laundry, repairs, ironing, or maintenance activities around the house or office benefits the metabolism, reducing risk by 10% or more of elevated metabolic biomarkers (cholesterol, triglycerides, waist circumference, metabolic syndrome).

You'll be surprised how quickly the time can add up as you take breaks in sitting. Every step you take counts and added together can make a difference.

Enhanced sitting

There is a variety of active sitting techniques that are simple yet provide benefits that counteract the negative reflex effects associated with sitting. Rocking in a rocking chair, or using foot-stimulating machines that vibrate, roll, or bathe the feet have been shown to reverse, eliminate, or improve some of the negative effects of sitting on the cardiovascular system.

TAKING BREAKS IN SITTING

If you take breaks from sitting, you might notice some of the following effects:

→ Re-setting of the metabolic mechanisms of the body, improving cholesterol, triglycerides, blood pressure, and blood-glucose levels as well as waistline size
→ Lessening of the strain on muscles, tendons, ligaments, and joints; decompression of pressure on the spine; lessening of discomfort and musculoskeletal pain; lessening of risk for falls and injury for all as well as mobility concerns later in life
→ Increase in blood flow to muscles, making them more receptive to insulin
→ Provision of more blood to the brain and heart
→ Burning more calories.

Enhanced walking

Enhance your walking experiences by considering where you walk and what's under your feet as you walk. Walking is more beneficial when you do it in a green, leafy setting or barefoot on a surface of rock, bamboo, or stone. Biomarkers and other measures of health are positively impacted when walking in enhanced circumstances when compared to those that aren't. Or, take a walk in a forest or green park, step/bounce on a mini-trampoline, or walk on a reflexology path or mat.

Reflex therapies

Perhaps you are familiar with reflexology, tai chi, and yoga. We consider them to be reflex therapies calling into action pressure sensors in the feet and/or the stretch and movement receptors of the postural muscles. Reflex therapies offer results unique among reflex techniques: pain reduction, improved gait, and lessened fear of falls in addition to impact on the metabolism. Also frequently noted is a sense of relaxation and calm.

SPARK YOUR CREATIVITY

While the reflex techniques we have noted have been studied with researched results, there are many other activities that have value as well. For example, you could stand to do your ironing rather than sit or ditch the golf cart and walk between holes. Get creative in being up and about.

The value of reflex techniques

The goal of the reflex "diet" is to add value to what you do throughout the day. Just as food has nutritional value, so too does what you do: the sitting, standing, walking, and moving about.

Mindfulness: realizing the value of what you do

This could be the best day of your body's life. As you follow the reflex "diet" be fully aware that you're building a better-functioning body as well as improving your overall health – be mindful of the changes you are making and how you are making them. As you implement the reflex "diet" and move through your day, you'll realize the importance of valuing what you're doing.

The goal of the reflex "diet" is to add value to what you do throughout the day.

With the reflex "diet", you'll be taking something that's been in the background and becoming aware, mindfully, of its value, so if you want to be successful in it, be mindful of what you're doing. What once was done without thought – sitting or standing – has the potential to shape you. What has been unconscious can be harnessed to make your body into the one you want. See page 29 for research about mindfulness.

Implementing your reflex "diet"

How do you add to your standing, walking, and moving time throughout the day? A goal is to substitute some of your sitting time with up-and-about activities. Another goal is to add purpose and focus to your day's activities by thinking about their "nutritional" value.

First, value when you are mobile since there's a benefit to realizing that what you do is having a positive impact. To discover how much time you are spending, time yourself or use an activity tracker such as a smartphone app or a reputable brand of tracking device. Next, think about your sitting time. Do you sit in one place for hours at a time at work, at home, or while traveling from place to place?

A goal is to substitute some of your sitting time with up-and-about activities.

From now on, aim towards sitting less and moving more. Implement your "recipe" for success as you sit for two hours less and move for two hours more than you currently do each day. You will see the benefits to your weight, metabolism, and more. You'll match the inner cave-dweller you with the life you're leading as a chair-dweller.

With these ingredients you are in control of your health and wellbeing. It's the reflex effects created by thousands of contractions of postural muscles and contacts to the pressure sensors of the feet with the right amount of time and timing. Adding this amount of movement to your day will provide enough activity down to the cellular level of the cave-dweller within to keep you healthier physically and mentally.

You're the boss, in charge, as you accentuate positive reflex activities and decrease negative reflex activities. You are the manager of your body. You decide where to put your resources to get to where you want to be. The result is the reflex "diet", a "menu" of techniques and a "recipe" for how much and how often to apply them.

CASE STUDY: CALORIE EXPENDITURE/MINDFULNESS

What happens when you become more aware of not only what
you do but also its value, and what it's doing for you? Weight loss
and blood-pressure reduction are the answers Dr. Ellen Langer of
Harvard University found when she worked with a group of hotel
maids about the value of their daily work.

In her study of 80 maids, one group of 40 was made aware of the
calories they expended during their day's work and that it more
than met the recommended half hour of daily exercise. One group
of 40 was not. "The researchers even provided specifics: 15 minutes
of scrubbing burns 60 calories, 15 minutes of vacuuming burns 50.
The basic message and the details were then posted in the maids'
hotels where the 44 women (in the aware group) worked, to serve
as reminders, while a control group was left in the dark."

Before the study 67% of the maids reported that they didn't
exercise. Their body shapes, measured by body fat and "waist-to-
hip" ratios, matched this perception, one that was different from
their actual amount of exercise. At the end of a month, those who
were aware lost an average of two pounds. In addition, their blood
pressure dropped an average of 10 points. Body fat and "waist-to-
hip" ratios improved as well. The maids who were not aware did
not have such results.

There were no reported changes in behavior, only in mind-set,
with the vast majority of the women now considering themselves
regular exercisers. Langer sees the study as a lesson in the
importance of mindfulness, long a subject of her research, and
which need not involve Buddhism or meditation, she stresses. "It's
about noticing new things; it's about engagement," she says.

2 Our chair-dwelling lifestyle

Our human story, physically, is about how we came to live our lives sitting in chairs and what this habit means to the cave-dweller inner "you" – reflexes automatically and unconsciously respond, with increased potential for damaging lifestyle conditions.

It's a chair-living world

How much you sit could very well answer many of the questions you have about why your body isn't behaving the way you want it to. Perhaps you've gained weight, have problems with cholesterol, or are being told you're pre-diabetic.

Our culture has led us to become chair-dwellers, but it's not too late to change things for the better. You can learn to use the central tool of that lifestyle, the chair, better, but it is important to realize that whatever your age, chair use accumulates with metabolic and other consequences.

Our current culture encourages us to sit: during our day's work; as we travel from place to place; during our evening's entertainment while engaged in television-watching, cell-phone chatting or texting, electronic game-playing, or computer use. As noted by one prolonged sitting researcher, Dr. James Levine, a Mayo Clinic endocrinologist, "With creativity, a person can eat, work, reproduce, play, shop and sleep without taking a step. Once enticed to the chair, we were stuck. Work and home alike: we do it sitting."

SITTING: THE NEW SMOKING

Sitting too much is called the "new smoking" for a reason, since prolonged sitting has surpassed smoking as a killer worldwide. Research shows that an hour of sitting shortens one's life by 22 minutes – the same amount of time as smoking two cigarettes. Over a lifetime, that's 1.8 years for men and 1.5 years for women – for each hour.

How did humankind come to a world of chair-living? We haven't been chair-sitting for that long in our evolutionary history. Researcher Eric Jensen notes that chairs have existed for only 500 generations, a mere blink of an eye in the evolutionary development of our physical bodies.

We haven't been chair-sitting for that long in our evolutionary history.

Our trek to prolonged sitting follows a trail of survival first with food gathering, then food producing (crop production), and then employment in jobs. As briefly summated from Dr. Levine's ideas, over eons "... hunter-gatherers became agriculturists, the Industrial Revolution moved us into factories and the technological revolution moved us behind desks."

The impact of sitting was first noted in a 1950s study of London bus drivers and conductors. When cardiac events were compared, it was the full-time sitters, the bus drivers, who suffered the most heart attacks. It was found that men who sat for long periods at work were twice as likely to develop heart disease as were men who moved around throughout the day.

Looking at sitting jobs from the 1970s onwards, researchers found that weight gain by Americans over the following 30 years resulted from fewer calories expended because sitting jobs replaced more active jobs.

The concern among researchers who have studied prolonged sitting? Unknown to us all: (1) health problems are caused by how long we sit and (2) we aren't taking the steps necessary to counteract them. And, chairs create "bad ergonomics and lack of movement", fostering for children bad behavior and impeding learning in the classroom; lessened performance in the workplace and, over a lifetime, risk for falls and impaired walking patterns in later life.

Moreover, prolonged sitting as a behavior impacts the bottom line of healthcare expenses, increasing the likelihood of a population needing more care for a host of lifestyle conditions. The cost of physical inactivity in the US is estimated to be $190 billion per year. The World Health Organization reports: "Physical inactivity has been identified as the fourth leading risk factor for global mortality (6% of deaths globally). Physical inactivity is estimated to be the main cause for approximately 21–25% of breast and colon cancers (90,000 cases per year in the US), 27% of diabetes and approximately 30% of ischemic heart disease burden."

Chair-dwelling habits: sitting time/screen time

So much of our lives are now lived sitting watching screens: television screens, computer device screens, and cell phones, or talking on cell phones. And there are huge ramifications. The main problem with screen-viewing is that we do it while we are sitting. Another problem is that it replaces time spent standing, walking, and moving about.

The nightly collapse

Ready to spend the evening with feet up in front of the television, hunkered down in front of the computer, or sprawled in a chair

THE BOTTOM LINE ON SITTING

By any measure, the story is the same: it's the lack of movement that is the issue. Not moving creates a negative physiological, reflexive response by the body.

THE EFFECTS OF AN EVENING OF SITTING

Think about how an evening of sitting can affect you, what researchers call "the four-hour threshold for leisure-time sitting".

↪ Twice the risk for obesity (3–4 hours for women; 3–6 hours for men)

↪ 113% increased risk of heart attack or stroke for men

↪ 80% increased risk of dying from cardiovascular disease

↪ Increased risk for men of abnormal metabolic indicators

↪ 94% higher odds for men and 54% for women of having metabolic syndrome, a condition predictive of diabetes and cardiovascular disease

↪ Double the levels of C-reactive protein, an indicator for cardiovascular disease and cancer

↪ Decrease in life span by 6 years for men and 7.2 years for women

or on the bed to chat on the cell phone, stream a video, or play an electronic game? Then welcome to the "nightly collapse".

It's a term that accurately describes what happens when many people, active at work or school all day, come home. Yes, it's a well-deserved break, but think about it: your body has its own schedule of metabolic needs and the evening, for many, consists of four or more hours of uninterrupted sitting time.

Your television is a "death threat"!

Watching television is the ultimate junk food for reflexes – if you're sitting as you watch. As with any seated activity, television-watching translates into muscles that don't move, don't consume fats and sugars, disrupting metabolism. Of all sedentary activities, however, television-viewing is particularly disruptive to physical and mental functions. It seems that television-viewing doesn't sufficiently keep the attention of the reflex system that runs metabolism and intellectual capabilities.

Study after study shows that television has more negative impact on the metabolic processes than other seated activities. Prolonged sitting while watching television results in increased risk for diabetes, obesity, cardiovascular disease (heart attack and stroke), Alzheimer's disease, and an increased risk for a shorter life span. In addition, television impacts mental processes and behavior in children.

RESEARCH ON SEDENTARY TV-WATCHING

As noted by researcher Dr. David Dunstan at the Baker IDI Heart and Diabetes Institute, a national research center in Victoria, Australia, "Television isn't lethal in and of itself; the real problem appears to be that sitting is the 'default position' ... Prolonged watching of television equals a lot of sitting, which invariably means there's an absence of muscle movement," Dunstan says. "If your muscles stay inactive for too long, it can disrupt your metabolism," he explains.

"The magnitude of this negative effect per 1 h(our) of sedentary TV time was about the same as the positive effect derived from 30 minutes of extra physical activity aimed at boosting health."

WATCHING TV CAN PILE ON THE POUNDS

In one study those who watched television for more than four hours a day were 46% more likely to die of any cause and 80% more likely to die of cardiovascular disease, compared to people who watched less than two hours a day. Compared to those who watched one hour of television a day, those who watched more than four hours were four time more likely to be overweight.

WHAT ONE HOUR OF TV CAN DO

The impact for each hour of television-viewing while sitting is shown as follows.

Weight: There was one-third of a pound weight gain for each hour of television-watching per day for those who watched between four and 11 hours. The average weight gain was 3.4 pounds per hour for participants over four years of age or a weight gain of nearly 17 pounds for those over 20 years of age

Cardiovascular disease: Risk of dying from cardiovascular disease increased by 18%

Cancer: Risk of dying from cancer increased by 9%

Longevity: Reduction in life expectancy by 22 minutes; 1.8 years over a lifetime for men and 1.5 years for women with information gathered over a six-year study

Metabolic syndrome: Associated with a 21% increase in risk for men, 26% increase in risk for women

Alzheimer's: 1.3 times increased risk for each hour per day of television-viewing during middle adulthood (ages 40 to 59) when combined with lack of other exercise and other hobbies

As noted by researcher Dr. Frank Hu of Harvard University: "Compared with other sedentary activities such as sewing, playing board games, reading, writing, and driving a car, TV-watching results in a lower metabolic rate."

Television-watching doesn't engage our bodies enough to prompt the metabolic systems into gear. Aside from physical, physiological disruptions related to sitting, it could be that television-watching is not that interesting for our brains. It doesn't give our brains enough to think about. Just as muscles improve with a workout, so too does the brain. Its workout is learning, something that is not provided by television-watching.

A view to kill

Researchers study television-watching to measure the impact of non-work sitting time, but they are now looking at other screens too – computer, cell phone, and tablets. One study found that Americans spend four and a half hours a day watching television and five and a quarter hours watching other screens. It's a matter of different screen, same health consequences.

RESEARCH ON SEDENTARY TV-WATCHING

According to American researcher Dr. Susan B. Sisson and colleagues of the Pennington Biomedical Research Center at Louisiana State University, who reviewed the sitting habits of 3,556 men and women, compared to men who sit for less than one hour per day watching television or using the computer outside work, those who sit more than four hours per day have:

➥ 94% higher or double the odds of having metabolic syndrome
➥ 88% higher odds of greater waist circumference
➥ 84% higher odds of low high-density lipoprotein cholesterol (HDLC)
➥ 55% higher odds of high blood pressure
➥ 32% higher odds of elevated glucose (2–3 hours/day)

For women the odds were different.

➥ 54% higher odds of having metabolic syndrome (for those who do not exercise)
➥ No association with higher odds of low high-density lipoprotein cholesterol (HDLC)

The researcher hypothesized that such a result is from women taking more breaks than men in sitting during their leisure time.

THE CELL-PHONE CONNECTION

The more time spent in cell-phone use, the poorer the cardiovascular health and the higher the body fat percentage. High-frequency users were also more likely to participate in further sedentary non-activities such as television-watching.

Computer use

While computer use may be more stimulating than television-watching, there are metabolic consequences. Men who spent more than four hours a day compared to two hours of non-work-related screen time (TV-viewing, surfing the internet, or playing video games) have a more than doubled (113%) increased risk of heart attack or stroke, a 50% increased risk of death, and are more likely to die by any cause.

Cell-phone use

We don't think of cell-phone use as contributing to the time we spend sitting every day, but it does. Frequent cell-phone users were less fit than infrequent cell-phone users according to one study. Just as with inactivity resulting from television-viewing, frequent cell-phone users were substituting phone use for active pastimes such as walking, exercise, and sports participation.

Are you a desk-chair potato?

"Desk-chair potato" is the newly coined term for those who spend most of the day sitting at work. As noted in *Men's Health* magazine, sedentary jobs have increased 83% since 1950. In the workplace of the 1980s, office workers spent 70% of their time sitting. Today it's 93%.

Women take more breaks than men in sitting during their leisure time, hypothesizes one researcher.

Results of such changes are reflected in barometers of health. A "significant portion" of the increase in body weight by men and women in the US, for example, is attributed to sedentary jobs. Researchers from the Pennington Biomedical Research Center at Louisiana State University looked at "trends in

THE EFFECTS OF LONG SITTING TIMES AT WORK

→ Walking at work increases creativity levels during and shortly after the walk, producing twice as many creative responses as when sitting

→ Sitting at work for 10 or more years doubled the risk of colon cancer and increased the risk of rectal cancer by 44%

→ A Chinese study found an increased risk of ovarian cancer for women who sat the most at work and while watching television at home

→ The risk for heart attack increases by 54% for people who sit for most of the day, according to researchers at Pennington Biomedical Research Center in Baton Rouge, LA

→ Sperm count is reduced for men who sit for over 2 hours at a time at work

→ Sitting at work for more than 95% of working time is associated with neck pain

→ More than half of taxi drivers in Beijing suffer from erectile dysfunction, a government survey has indicated

→ Each 2-hour per day increment in sitting at work was associated with a 7% increase in risk for diabetes for women

→ Each 2-hour per day increment in sitting at work was associated with a 5% increase in risk for obesity for women

occupational physical activity" over time and found that both men and women expend 100 calories less a day on the job. This "change in occupation-related daily energy expenditure... closely matched the actual change in weight for 40–50-year-old men and women."

Aside from the metabolic dis-regulation potential of on-the-job sitting, pain and musculoskeletal distress result from chair time at work. Researcher Eric Jensen notes that: "The typical office

A SEDENTARY LIFESTYLE FOR OUR KIDS
Children and teenagers sit all day at school and they are often transported from place to place by car. They sit more during their leisure-time activities, playing passive video games, using computers, texting, talking on cell phones, and watching television.

worker has more musculoskeletal problems than any other industry-sector worker, including construction, metal industry and transport workers. ... One researcher's conclusion: Sitting is as much an occupational risk as lifting heavy weights on the job."

Just as smoking used to be an issue in the workplace, so too is prolonged sitting. Research shows that sedentary jobs increase the risk for multiple lifestyle conditions. It also shows that sitting increases risk for abnormal biomarkers, indicators of risk for lifestyle conditions. At the same time, many employers are pushing employees to take more responsibility for maintaining their own health, measured frequently by metabolic biomarkers. Yet the very same seated jobs create abnormal metabolic biomarkers for blood pressure, weight, cholesterol, and more.

Just as smoking used to be an issue in the workplace, so too is prolonged sitting.

Where is the the balance between employer expectations for health responsibility and employee job requirements that include prolonged sitting? Can employers expect employees to be responsible for their own health concerns which are created by the very demands of their employment?

Why are some children so fat?
Those who try to figure out the reasons for childhood obesity or why children do poorly or behave badly in school might do well to consider the time they spend sitting down when they could be active. Research shows a direct connection between children's sitting time and "decreased fitness, poor self-esteem, weak academic performance, obesity and increased aggression".

RESEARCH ON CHILDREN WATCHING TV

Canadian researchers observed children watching television and measured their physiological biomarkers. After two to seven hours of uninterrupted sitting, there is evidence "that it is enough to increase (subjects') blood sugar, to decrease their good cholesterol and to have a real impact on their health", according to researcher Travis Saunders of the Children's Hospital of Eastern Ontario Research Institute in Ottawa.

When compared to children who watched between zero and two hours' TV a day, children who watched more than five hours a day were at 4.6 times more likely to be overweight. Harvard researchers S. L. Gortmaker et al. estimated that 60% of the "overweight incidence" was linked to television-watching. Further research showed additional concerns related to children and TV-viewing. An analysis of 232 studies of sedentary behavior in children with a total of 983,840 participants found that more than two hours per day of TV-viewing form a critical time barrier, resulting in: reduced physical and psychosocial health; increased weight/BMI; "... decreased fitness; lowered scores for self-esteem and pro-social behavior and decreased academic achievement"; and increased risk for metabolic syndrome and cardiovascular conditions.

"Canadian children and youth spend 62% of their waking hours in sedentary pursuits, with six to eight hours per day of screen time as the average for school-aged kids," said Dr. Mark Tremblay of the University of Ottawa, Canada. "Lower levels of sedentary behaviour are consistently associated with improved body composition, cardiorespiratory and musculoskeletal fitness, academic achievement and even self-esteem."

RISK FACTORS OF SCREEN GAME-PLAYING

Research found console/video game-playing by teenagers, for example, to be associated with increased risk for cardiovascular biomarkers, including elevated blood pressure and fats in overweight teenagers' blood.

RESEARCH ON TEENAGER BEHAVIOR

Spanish researcher, David Martinez-Gomez, states that older teenage males (16–19-year-olds) are among the most sedentary of any age group, second only to senior citizens. Teenage sedentary behavior "raise(s) significant concerns about the early development of (teenagers) behaviour [sic] patterns and body habits, attributes that may significantly increase the risk of major chronic diseases (particularly type two diabetes, cardiovascular disease, and breast and colon cancer). While these diseases may not manifest themselves until later in adult life, it seems that not only the behavioural [sic] basis, but also the biological precursors for these chronic diseases may be established during adolescence."

For children, prolonged sitting problems include those associated with physical development, risk for early-onset lifestyle conditions, as well as problems with behavior and performance in school. The stage is set for lifestyle conditions later in life – lifetime sitting habits begin when young.

How does sitting impact some adults?

Sitting impacts quality of life as well as how well you age. Health concerns echoing in later years include Alzheimer's, walking instability, diabetes, heart disease, and metabolic disorders. Consider how much uninterrupted sitting time impacts metabolism. An Australian study showed that more than

THE GYM MAY NOT BE ENOUGH

If you're an adult who thinks that your exercise program keeps you fit, think again. "Consider this: We've become so sedentary that 30 minutes a day at the gym may not do enough to counteract the detrimental effects of eight, nine, or ten hours of sitting," says Dr. Genevieve Healy, "That's one big reason so many women still struggle with weight, blood sugar, and cholesterol woes despite keeping consistent workout routines."

two hours per day of television-viewing increased: abnormal concentrations of cholesterol, triglycerides, and other fats in the blood; risk of insulin resistance (linked to diabetes and heart disease) and obesity.

The more you sit, the bigger your waistline is likely to be.

The more you sit, the bigger your waistline is likely to be. The more you sit, the greater the increase in your risk for obesity. Every two uninterrupted hours of television-watching in the evening increases the risk for obesity – by 23%. Every two hours of television-viewing increases the risk of cardiovascular disease by 15%, according to an analysis of four studies from the US, Europe, and Australia, with a total of 34,253 participants, conducted by Dr. Frank Hu of Harvard and Danish researcher Anders Grontved.

Metabolic dysfunction is one of the mechanisms thought to be at work linking prolonged sitting and increased risk for endometrial, ovarian, and prostate cancer. Some 30% of colon cancer and 21% of breast cancers may be due to physical inactivity. Those who worked at a sedentary job for ten or more years increased their risk for colon cancer by 44%.

Those who are overweight at 50 have an increased risk of earlier cognitive decline. Those who are overweight with two metabolic biomarkers (high blood pressure, blood glucose, triglycerides or low "good" cholesterol) at age 50 have the cognitive decline of a healthy individual seven years older. Prolonged sitting impacts each of these elements. Those whose primary "hobby" in adult years is television-watching have a 250% increased risk of Alzheimer's. The groundwork for musculoskeletal problems later in life is created during earlier years. Sitting too much strains tendons and ligaments as well as placing stress on the spine.

How does sitting impact some seniors?

Among the elderly, those least physically active during the day are more likely to develop Alzheimer's. Even activities like cooking, washing dishes, playing cards, and moving a wheelchair as well as rocking in a rocking chair were beneficial.

According to Dr. Aron Buchman's research among participants averaging 82 years old, those who are physically inactive are 2.3 times more likely to develop Alzheimer's. "… Rocking-chair therapy could become an important treatment tool for the approximately 1.6 million people in US nursing homes, more than half of whom suffer from some form of dementia."

3 The cave-dweller within

The cave-dweller within us contends with a life doing very different things from those for which the human body was designed. Our ancient ancestors were a great deal more active than we are now. They spent their day on their feet, whereas we spend our day mostly sitting down, whether traveling in a vehicle, sitting at a desk, or relaxing in front of the TV.

You don't see what goes on in the inner "you" to make your day happen. Postural muscles and pressure sensors communicate with the inner "you" about your body being in motion – or not. The inner "you" responds in a coordinated activity that includes metabolism, the musculoskeletal system, the veins and arteries of the circulatory system, and makes calculations within the nervous system and brain. Sit too much and the body's reflex system fails to receive enough of a workout through the day: the internal "you", brought to life by activity, suffers *It's all about stimulus and response.* from lack of stimulation. It's all about stimulus and response. Without sufficient stimulus, the metabolic response is thrown into disarray, arteries clog with fats, insulin builds in the bloodstream, appetite regulators are thrown off, weight gain occurs, and circulation slows. Pain creeps into joints and muscles.

The body metabolizes fats and sugars as well as performing other activities appropriate to the activity of sitting.

Unfortunately, this is not what our bodies are designed to do. When we sit too much, many of these processes shut down. The net result is increased risk for lifestyle conditions, cognitive decline, and lessened abilities to move well. Included are risks for cardiovascular disease, stroke, heart attack, diabetes, obesity, cognition as well as, later in life, Alzheimer's, hastened cognitive decline, dementia, walking difficulties, and falls.

Discussed in this chapter is what happens to the cave-dweller within living a chair-dweller lifestyle and why it happens that our time spent sitting, standing, and walking shapes our health and risk for lifestyle conditions.

Metabolism disrupted

A day spent sitting disrupts metabolism in a cascading series of events. Muscles not active in standing and walking mean that fats and sugars remain in the bloodstream. The regulators of fats and sugars become dysfunctional and "resistant" to future proper regulation. With metabolism failing to operate efficiently, risk for obesity, cardiovascular ill health, type-two diabetes, and other lifestyle conditions increase.

"Just like exercise, prolonged sitting has distinct physiological effects. But unlike exercise, sitting has unhealthy effects."

But what about exercise? Can it help? Yes, but, as one researcher notes, the average person can't exercise enough to have an impact. This is because the metabolic processes and types of muscles used as we stand and walk are actually a part of the metabolic, muscular, and nervous system, which isn't used during exercise. Physical inactivity researcher Dr. Marc Hamilton of the Pennington Biomedical Research Laboratory states that the gene that causes heart disease becomes "worse" with sitting and "better" only with "contractile activity" in postural muscles used while standing or walking.

Re-setting your metabolism

The more you move, the more effective your metabolism. The more you sit, the less effective your metabolism. For those who don't exercise, some 90% of calories are utilized in sitting, standing, or walking around. Making the decision about what to do with your time and energy can determine the imprint of the chair-dwelling lifestyle on the inner cave-dwelling "you".

Substituting sitting time with up-and-about time around the house or office can substantially increase resistance to weight gain and improve metabolism.

Making the decision about what to do with your time and energy can determine the imprint of the chair-dwelling lifestyle on the inner cave-dwelling "you".

Metabolism is all about energy. Think about the fact that leg muscles don't move as you sit. As a result, fuels – fats and sugars – circulating in the bloodstream, are not utilized. Because fats and sugar are not used by muscles, there is a higher concentration of them in the blood and disarray in metabolism results. This disarray creates abnormal levels of fats (triglycerides and "good" HDL cholesterol) and sugar (glucose). Impacted as well is blood pressure as arteries lined with fats that are not metabolized narrow and cause the heart to beat more. The waistline increases in size as well.

Taken together, the measurements for these five (triglycerides, cholesterol, glucose, blood pressure, and waistline size) serve as indicators for metabolic syndrome. An individual with metabolic syndrome has abnormal measures in three of the five areas. Those with metabolic syndrome are at increased risk for the lifestyle conditions of cardiovascular disease, diabetes, obesity, and more.

WHAT IS YOUR "FAT VACUUM WITHIN"?

The fat vacuum within is the enzyme lipoprotein lipase. The term "vacuum for fat", coined by researcher Marc Hamilton, notes the action of lipoprotein lipase to facilitate fat uptake from the bloodstream as we stand and walk.

Your fat vacuum

What happens to your metabolism when the chair-dwelling
you sits more than mandated by the cave-dweller inner "you"?
For one thing, your fat vacuum stays silent.
A fat vacuum within? And it's possible to
communicate with this vacuum and get it
going? Sounds good, you're thinking, where
do I sign up?

*You activate your fat
vacuum every time you
stand up and/or walk.*

Actually, you activate your fat vacuum every time you stand up
and/or walk. Standing or walking engages the fat vacuum within
as your foot's pressure sensors and body's postural muscles are
at work and signal the need for fuel, the fats and sugars that are
circulating in the bloodstream.

RESEARCH ON FATS AND LPL IN THE BLOODSTREAM

Researchers were aware that prolonged sitting leads to higher
levels of fats appearing in the bloodstream, but they didn't know
how or why. Fortunately, the work of researcher Dr. Marc Hamilton
created such an understanding. He found that mice whose legs
were inactive for one day experienced a change in levels of an
enzyme in the bloodstream important to metabolizing fats. The
levels of the enzyme lipoprotein lipase (LPL) were one-tenth of
that for active mice. Humans share that enzyme with mice.

Hamilton's research with mice shows that the fat vacuum is active
only when leg muscles are being flexed as we stand or walk, but
luckily activating your fat vacuum is as easy as standing up and/
or walking. Especially as you walk, muscles are contracting and
relaxing, activating LPL, and fat is being vacuumed from your
bloodstream.

Chair-dwelling creates a dis-regulation of the fat vacuum. Our bodies are designed to process fat on a schedule that involves standing and moving about for most of the day. Sit for a few hours and the fat vacuum starts to turn off. Sit all day and 50% less of the fat vacuum is available to metabolize the fat, according to researcher Dr. James Levine of the Mayo Clinic who, incidentally, coined the term "chair-living". Why the fat vacuum goes awry gives a clue as to how we can help our bodies work better, achieving all sorts of weight and health goals.

Cellular level

Prolonged sitting has an impact down to the molecular level. The ability to process the fat circulating in the bloodstream gets thrown off as we sit for a prolonged time.

Higher levels of lipoprotein lipase are an indicator that we're up and about, of postural muscles at work. Lipoprotein lipase is important to breaking down triglycerides, HDL cholesterol, and other metabolic risk factors in the bloodstream. Abnormalities in lipoprotein lipase function, lower levels indicating a lower level of moving about, are linked to a myriad lifestyle conditions: atherosclerosis, obesity, Alzheimer's, metabolic syndrome, and a low HDL ("good fat")/high LDL ("bad fat") condition associated with diabetes, insulin resistance.

Prime your sugar pump

Movement is fueled not only by fats but by sugar as well. Sugar moves from the bloodstream into the muscles aided by the hormone insulin also circulating in the bloodstream. Use of postural muscles, contracting and relaxing as we stand and walk, increases blood flow to muscles, so they're more receptive to insulin. Your brain runs on glucose as well, consuming 60% of the body's glucose when it is at rest. The brain requires a continuous supply of glucose as it has no way to store fuel.

Leg muscles that don't move as you sit for a prolonged period results in sugar remaining in the blood. The increase of sugar in the blood is seen by the inner "you" as a need for more insulin

ACTIVATE YOUR SUGAR PUMP

Taking frequent breaks increases blood flow to muscles. Also, activating the enzyme LPL by moving helps prevent insulin resistance. Those who take the most breaks in sitting have the best profiles for both sugar and fat metabolism. A 15-minute walking break after eating or a 2-minute walking break every 20 minutes helps normalize blood-sugar levels.

to metabolize the increasing sugar. What follows is chaos in the metabolism of sugar as muscles are perceived as resisting the "uptake" of sugar or "insulin resistance". Eventually the pancreas fails to produce enough insulin and type-two diabetes results.

How much does sitting too much impact the metabolism of sugar? Research shows that one day of sitting reduces insulin action by 39%. Indicators of risk for diabetes, impaired metabolism of sugars (insulin resistance) and increased weight around the middle, are increased by prolonged sitting. Such disruption of sugar metabolism impacts weight. Some 80% of Americans with type-two diabetes are overweight or obese.

Sitting and waist size

Did you realize that a large waist size is an indicator for how well your metabolism is working? Or that walking and standing may have more to do with your waistline size than exercise directed at reducing the waistline?

A large waist size along with cholesterol, triglyceride, and C-reactive protein levels are indicators of cardio-metabolic function and cardiovascular risk. Prolonged sitting periods are associated with a larger waistline. Even among those who sit for long periods, the more breaks in sitting, the smaller the waist.

Blood pressure, up and down with sitting

There are multiple causes for high blood pressure, but physical inactivity is among them. When we stand or walk, postural muscles of the calves contract and relax. The veins located within them compress and decompress, pumping blood from the extremities, helping return it to the brain and heart. As we sit, the heart pumps harder to compensate for the lack of movement by leg muscles. With prolonged sitting, high blood pressure is the result.

In general, for those who sit too much this results in higher blood pressure. Men who sit more than four hours per day during their off time have 55% higher blood pressure.

For many of us, sitting is a relaxing activity. But not for everyone. For half of the women in one study, 20 minutes of sitting had a profound effect on blood pressure, going up instead of down. The researcher hypothesized that their hearts worked harder to return blood from the extremities because of a lack of muscle tone in the legs.

The importance of adequate circulation is that it provides the nutrients of glucose and oxygen to the brain. The brain consumes 60% of the body's glucose and 25% of its oxygen when the body is at rest. Lack of profusion of blood to the brain is suspected as increasing the risk for cognitive decline, dementia, and Alzheimer's. Also pain in the legs and thrombosis can result.

Re-set your appestat, re-boot your metabolism

How do we know we're full and don't need to eat more? This is a key component in gaining weight. Our body tells us whether we're full or not through the appestat, its natural appetite control. More than that, the biomarkers circulating in the blood to indicate hunger also signal information about metabolism and are linked to cardiovascular disease, obesity, Alzheimer's, and other disorders.

Prolonged sitting sets off a chain of events leading to dis-regulation of the body's appestat.

Prolonged sitting sets off a chain of events leading to dis-regulation of the body's appestat – its natural appetite control.

The result is eating more food than necessary to move through the day, in other words, gaining weight. The appestat in the brain, the hypothalamus, makes calculations about our need to eat. Such a need is a survival mechanism serving to make sure we eat to fuel our activities. The appestat tracks a protein, leptin, and the hormone insulin as they circulate in the bloodstream. Insulin provides reports about the availability of sugar (a short-term fuel) and leptin provides information about fat (a long-term fuel) to be utilized in the movement of muscles.

As we stand or walk, movement is fueled as sugar (glucose) moves from the bloodstream into the muscles, aided by the hormone insulin. The amount of insulin in the bloodstream serves as an indicator of fuel use by the muscles. The circulation of insulin in the bloodstream is continually monitored by the appestat of the brain, which acts on such information to regulate other hormones related to feelings of fullness in the stomach and intestines to dampen or increase the appetite.

As noted, leptin is a biomarker for cardiovascular disease, obesity, Alzheimer's, and other disorders. It circulates in the bloodstream, having been released from fat cells as an indicator of how much triglyceride, a fat used to fuel movement of muscles, is being stored. A high amount of leptin in the bloodstream indicates that there is enough fuel stored and eating more is not necessary. It serves to suppress the appetite.

Leptin and insulin resistance

As we move – or don't move – reflex actions take place that determine how well our appestat mechanism works. As we walk or stand, the "uptake" of fats and sugars from the bloodstream by muscles at work happens automatically and unconsciously. If we sit too much, the appestat mechanism goes awry.

If we sit too much, the appestat mechanism goes awry.

Insulin resistance happens when insulin builds up in the bloodstream as muscles don't move often enough. Similarly, increases in leptin levels create leptin resistance.

LEPTIN IMPLICATIONS

High levels of the hormone leptin were associated with lower rates of Alzheimer's disease in a study appearing in *The Journal of the American Medical Association.*

If confirmed, researchers say the findings could have important implications in the search for effective therapies to prevent and treat the disease.

As noted by Dr. Louis J. Aronne, "... in most cases, obesity is associated with leptin resistance – as leptin levels rise in association with increased fat reserves, fail-safe mechanisms built into the body reduce the effectiveness of leptin signaling." Leptin resistance occurs. The net result of insulin resistance and leptin resistance is an appetite gone awry, an appestat unable to regulate appropriately.

Inflammation

Inflammation is thought to be one pathway linking prolonged sitting with risk for cardiovascular disease and cancer. C-reactive protein in the bloodstream is an indicator of inflammation. Inflammation can play a role in hardening of the arteries, considered to be the cause of half of all strokes. Inflammation results from chronic accumulation of fats in arteries and chronic inflammation arising from several sources can predispose an individual to cancer.

Research shows that the more the sedentary behavior, the worse the indicators for inflammation and cardiovascular risk. A British study found that those who sit for more than four hours per day during non-work screen time (TV-viewing, surfing the internet, or playing video games) have the indicator C-reactive protein circulating in their bloodstreams with a level approximately two times higher than those who sit for less than two hours. Those who spent the most non-work time in front of a screen (more than six hours) had levels three times higher.

It's in the way you walk – or don't

Just as our metabolisms are designed to work as we stand and move, our musculoskeletal systems are intended to hold us upright in a standing position – not a sitting one.

Standing is the natural position to properly distribute our weight. The natural curve of the spine works to hold us upright as we move. A stable base for standing and walking is created as hips and lower back are held in place by a group of muscles called the hip flexors.

Sitting for too long creates musculoskeletal stress and, over time, dysfunction. The natural curve of the spine is distorted, no longer holding us upright against gravity, as intended, requiring other muscles of the back to work to hold it in place.

Chair-sitting literally re-shapes the body. Muscles and, over a lifetime, bone itself, come to take a shape commensurate with chair-sitting rather than standing up or walking. When your postural muscles are quiet, losing their tone, they become more proficient at sitting and less proficient at standing and walking. The result is the changing postural profile of middle age followed by aging, and then aged. Abilities to stand and walk are compromised, which is understandable over a lifetime, as they have been under-practiced and under-used.

Among other results, especially among office workers, is physical discomfort and musculoskeletal pain – neck pain, upper-back pain and, by one estimate, a tripling of lower-back pain among women since 1990. Headaches and numbness in limbs are reported. One expert notes that "distortion of the natural curve of the spine during too much sitting leads to chronic pain at some time in the lives of 80% of Americans."

Standing is the natural position to properly distribute our weight.

Half of newly hired workers whose jobs included 15 or more hours of computer use a week reported neck or shoulder and

RESEARCH ON SITTING AND OCCUPATIONAL RISK

Researcher Eric Jensen notes that "The typical office worker has more musculoskeletal problems than any other industry-sector worker, including construction, metal industry, and transport workers." One researcher's conclusion states: "Sitting is as much an occupational risk as lifting heavy weights on the job."

hand or arm musculoskeletal symptoms by the end of their first year of employment, as described in an Emory University study.

Particularly impacted as we sit too much are the hamstring muscles and hip flexors. Lift your knee and then lower it. You've just utilized these muscles, which are central to taking each footstep. Intended to shorten and lengthen as we move, they remain shortened and they tighten as we sit.

Over time, such tightening results in loss of flexibility with the lower back becoming a less stable platform when one stands or walks. Range of motion is limited and risk for injury increases.

Compromised is what one therapist calls "movement competence", impacting performance and potential for injury while moving through the day or playing sports. For all of us, it's an increased potential for mis-step and injury. For the weekend athlete, it's abilities to hit the golf ball or make that jump shot that have diminished. For the elderly,

A risk of falling may be an early indicator of Alzheimer's.

it's decreasing abilities to walk well and risks for mobility.

Concerns about aging

A loss of flexibility in the lower back creates concerns about aging. "Flexibility, particularly in your lower body, is a key determinant in how well you age, including your risk of falling and your ability to get around." A risk of falling may be an early indicator of Alzheimer's. One researcher found

RESEARCH ON COGNITIVE DECLINE

Walking abilities are tied to cognitive decline. One Japanese researcher measured senior citizens' abilities to walk their fastest over 18 feet. He found the slower the walk, the more the signs of dementia. "Our research found that gait velocity (speed) was significantly decreased as the severity of dementia symptoms increased," he notes: "Gait should no longer be considered a simple, automatic, motor activity that is independent of cognition. They are linked."

Italian researchers measured elderly study participants walking initially and then 15 months later. They found that study participants with fewer steps per minute, slower speed, and shorter distance between steps, the more the decline in cognition, memory and decision making "... experienced significantly larger declines in global cognition, memory and executive function".

more than double the risk for a fall over an eight-month period among study participants who had PET scans showing signs of amyloid, an early indicator of Alzheimer's.

How sitting too much affects your appearance

Sitting too much influences not just health but also the way you look. For women, think big behind, protruding stomach, and hunched back as muscles, hip flexors, and hamstrings are unnaturally utilized. The buttocks are thrust out as the pelvis is pulled forward as muscles linking leg and hips tighten. The stomach protrudes as abdominal muscles, normally balancing leg/hip muscle activity, weaken as they remain inactive during sitting. A hunched back results from sitting too much.

Also influencing a big behind is what researchers found when they manipulated fat cells to remain sedentary for long periods

BIOMARKER AND INDICATOR SUMMARY

CONDITION	BIOMARKERS AND INDICATORS
Cardiovascular disease, stroke, heart attack	Waist circumference, HDL ("good" cholesterol), blood pressure, higher glucose levels, C-reactive protein, triglycerides, insulin resistance, abnormal levels of lipoprotein lipase
Weight	Triglycerides, HDL ("good" cholesterol), blood pressure, leptin, abnormalities in lipoprotein lipase function
Cognition, productivity	Glucose, circulation (of blood to the brain)
Cognitive impairment	Dis-regulation of metabolism, obesity, gait abnormalities
Dementia	Risk factors: high blood pressure, higher blood-sugar levels, diabetes, obesity, gait abnormalities
Alzheimer's	Risk factors: physical inactivity/sedentary behavior, factors related to inactivity – midlife obesity, midlife hypertension, and diabetes, depression, higher blood-sugar levels, abnormal levels of lipoprotein lipase
Cancer	Metabolic dysfunction (waist circumference, insulin resistance/glucose), leptin dysfunction, and C-reactive protein, body mass index
Diabetes	Higher than normal blood-glucose levels, insulin, physical inactivity, obesity, diabetes in the family
Metabolic syndrome	Biomarkers (3 of the 5): triglycerides, HDL ("good" cholesterol), glucose, blood pressure, and waist size
Mental clarity	Return of blood from the extremities and circulation of blood to the heart. The nutrients of glucose and oxygen provided to the brain
Musculoskeletal system	Muscles, tendons, and ligaments important to gait, cognition, and maintaining a stable base for walking

of time. The fat cells stretched and "produced nearly 50% more liquid fat than regular fat cells". They hypothesize that the fat cells are influenced not only by calorie consumption but also by the mechanical environment of being stretched as one sits.

To sum up

The cave-dweller within each of us faces risks of lifestyle conditions as the biomarkers and other indicators are shaped by a chair-dwelling lifestyle. The chart on the facing page is a summary of lifestyle conditions, biomarkers, and indicators linked to sitting too much.

4 Your reflex "diet"

What kinds of body and mind do you want? You can leave it to chance and hope for the best or you can design a new "you" with the reflex "diet". It's a life-assurance policy. By investing in, and planning to add, moving to your day, you protect your body and mind.

The chair-dwelling lifestyle has an impact on the cave-dwelling inner "you". The impact is quantifiable. A particular amount of uninterrupted sitting time has a particular impact. The same applies to standing and walking time. This is where the reflex "diet" comes in. We have documented how much sitting, standing, and moving time create the body and mind you want.

You can become an active chair-dweller, making decisions about sitting and moving, taking control of the direction your body and mind are going.

What the reflex "diet" can do for you

Giving your standing and walking reflexes the workout they need every day is a component of good health. Nutrition and exercise are important to health, but there is no substitute for being up and about.

You can become an active chair-dweller.

Getting up and moving about the home or office more not only expends more calories but also builds toward re-setting reflex mechanisms thrown off by prolonged sitting. These metabolic and other mechanisms are the basic indicators of progression toward lifestyle conditions such as obesity, diabetes, stroke, heart attack, cognitive decline, and more.

THE REFLEX "DIET" WILL IMPACT:

→ Weight
→ Metabolism
→ Lifestyle conditions
→ Longevity

→ Mental acuity
→ Musculoskeletal
   comfort and flexibility
→ Mobility

The reflex "diet" provides you with a road map to impact the above mechanisms (see box), your calorie expenditure, overall health, and the potential for resulting lifestyle conditions.

Maybe you're seeking a general goal such as wellness, brain power, productivity, or longevity. Perhaps you're at a crossroads with a lifestyle condition, a hereditary predisposition, or a current concern, or you're heading for a lifestyle condition.

The "recipe" for success

When you're up and about as much as intended by the body's evolutionary design, the reflex mechanisms that manage the body for us are able to go about their work in a healthy way. The minimum daily requirement for a healthy "you" is what is called the "recipe for success": move two hours more a day and take breaks every 20 minutes for two minutes.

In other words, stand, walk, and move for two hours more a day than you do currently. Time spent taking breaks counts towards the two additional hours a day of being up and about. If you can't take a break from sitting every 20 minutes, take one once an hour for at least five minutes.

Targeting your health

The reflex "diet" helps you work toward your health by giving you targets for decreasing your sitting time and increasing your active time. Reflex techniques – sitting time, standing up, moving about, taking breaks in sitting – all re-set reflex mechanisms. When practiced over time, change is created and risk of lifestyle conditions is lessened.

MOVING TWO HOURS MORE A DAY

Results in:
- Better profiles for metabolic biomarkers
- Better profile for C-reactive protein
- Expenditure of more calories
- Re-setting of the body's appestat
- Lessened risks for diabetes, cancer, cardiovascular disease, metabolic syndrome, obesity, diabetes, musculoskeletal stress

Lifestyle conditions impacted:
- Cardiovascular disease, stroke, heart attack
- Weight
- Cognition, productivity
- Dementia and Alzheimer's
- Cancer
- Diabetes
- Metabolic syndrome

Adding movement to your day and considering your sitting time will help you build a healthier life and levels of the basic indicators for the progression of lifestyle disorders.

Create your reflex "diet" by considering the value of your efforts among the array of reflex techniques noted in Chapters 5–9. Some techniques may be a part of your daily routine now, so you'll be aware of their value. Other techniques may present an opportunity to add to your day.

Getting started on your reflex "diet"

Implement the basic reflex "diet" by first considering how to go about standing, walking, and moving for two hours more a day than you do currently as well as taking a break in sitting every 20 minutes for two minutes.

TAKING TWO-MINUTE BREAKS EVERY 20 MINUTES

Results in:

→ Lower blood pressure

→ Impact on glucose, insulin, with insulin resistance

→ Re-sets muscles, tendons, and ligaments

→ Lessened risks for diabetes, cancer, cardiovascular disease, metabolic syndrome, diabetes, musculoskeletal stress

→ Expenditure of more calories

Lifestyle conditions impacted:

→ Cardiovascular disease, stroke, heart attack

→ Cancer

→ Mental clarity

→ Diabetes

→ Metabolic syndrome

→ Musculoskeletal system

Measuring and moving

How do you know you're moving two hours more a day? Start by measuring how much time you move during a day. One easy way to do this is to measure the steps you take using a wearable fitness tracker. Once you have a baseline, add steps. An hour more a day represents approximately 2,000 steps taken during activities around the home or office. Consider the benefits of taking steps from 7,500 a day to 10,000 a day. See Chapter 7 (page 96).

Start by creating increments of moving. A sedentary person takes 3,000 steps a day. The average office worker takes 5,000 steps a day. Give yourself time to build your up-and-about time. Consider adding a few steps here and there throughout the day. Take the long way around instead of the short cut as you go from place to place at work or walking directly to the item you intend to purchase at the store. Small amounts of active time add up. As noted by Dr. Alpa Patel, standing or walking for five minutes every hour results in an hour of non-sitting time over a 12-hour period during the day. Taking a two-minute break every 20 minutes or six minutes every hour results in a total of being up and about for one hour and 12 minutes over a 12-hour day.

What reflex techniques to use

The techniques of the reflex "diet" are more than sitting down, standing up, and walking around. Reflex techniques have a value. How much time spent in which activities will create for you the reflex "diet" to achieve your goals? See Chapters 5–9.

Your break strategy

Consider your breaks. You will probably have a work strategy and a home strategy.

Plan to move throughout your day. This gives your metabolism the workout best for the inner cave-dweller "you".

At work a two-minute break every 20 minutes has been shown to be especially beneficial for relieving muscular discomfort for those whose work includes sitting at the computer. Even a one-minute standing break creates relief and has been shown not to interrupt productivity. A five-minute break in sitting every hour is considered necessary.

While not all employees are free to move around at all times, some employers encourage movement. At Google, for example, some desks automatically rise every hour to remind employees to move. At Cessna Aircraft a tone sounds to signal employees to move about. Other employers install computer software that reminds employees to get up and move about.

How to time breaks

If you need to establish 20 minutes of sitting and then a two-minute break, how do you know 20 minutes has gone by and then two minutes? There are timing options ranging from an egg timer to smart phone apps to reminders on a computer.

TECHNIQUE CONSIDERATIONS

Decide which technique will:

➡ Meet your goals

➡ Match the time, money, and effort you can afford

➡ Suit you

➡ Be good value (as it helps you get to where you want to be)

If you're at home watching television, commercials pop up at regular intervals. As a commercial comes on, stand up, move about, or step in place, and then sit down again when the commercial is over. As noted by one researcher, you'll be doing more for yourself since the commercials last longer than two minutes and appear more frequently than every 20 minutes (see Chapter 6).

Targeting a lifestyle health concern

Changing sitting and moving habits allows you to target a lifestyle health concern. Consider, for example, the potential for increasing cardiovascular health and decreasing the risk of cardiovascular disease. Lowering one's blood pressure by a specific amount lessens one's risk for stroke and coronary heart disease (see page 144). Researchers in prolonged sitting have found decreased sitting time and increased active time can lower blood pressure. Choose from among reflex techniques to consider your reflex diet to target your health concern (see Chapters 5–9).

A friend created her own program. She took breaks by visiting the drinking fountain, coffee room, rest room, another part of the building, or fetching something from her car.

There are multiple reflex techniques that contribute to lessening blood pressure and cardiovascular risk.

➡ Researchers found walking 10,000 steps a day for 12 weeks lowered sustained diastolic blood pressure by eight points.

➡ Two-minute breaks in sitting every 20 minutes over seven hours was associated with systolic and diastolic blood pressure lowered by three points compared to that of uninterrupted sitting.

➥ When compared to study participants who walked on a normal surface three times a week for 45 minutes over four months, those who walked on a cobblestone mat experienced a lower diastolic blood pressure (4.75 points).

➥ Study participants who practiced yoga for four weeks to 12 months: "demonstrated a 4.9% to 24.2% decline in diastolic blood pressure and a 2.6% to 21.3% decline in systolic blood pressure ..."

➥ Wearing Kenkoh massage sandals for four hours while moving about reduced systolic blood pressure (12%), diastolic blood pressure (6%), as well as lowered pulse rate (18%), compared to those who wore smooth-soled sandals.

➥ One hour of tai chi three times per week for 12 weeks was associated with significant improvements in systolic and diastolic blood pressure.

➥ Watching television one less hour a day resulted in a "diastolic blood pressure difference of 0.7 points in men and 0.5 in women ... (which) could result in a risk reduction of CHD (cardiovascular heart disease) and stroke of 2.5 and 4% respectively."

➥ Those who take the most breaks in sitting "showed smaller waistlines (1½") and reduced levels of C-reactive protein, a marker for heart disease indicating inflammation."

To maximize your time and minimize your effort you'll want to find opportunities to move around more.

Design your reflex "diet"

So, what's a person to do? Stand at work during the day and then again in the living room all evening? Those who have tried this for a month report that it is boring and results in sore feet. No, you should design a routine that works for you.

To maximize your time and minimize your effort you'll want to: find opportunities to move around more, make plans to move throughout the day, set the scene by putting in place the tools you need, and establish your goals for what you to accomplish.

Planning for success

Plan to help your inner cave-dweller live better in a chair-dwelling world. The reflex "diet" is about forming habits that will make a difference in how you feel and maximize the way your body works. Chairs are a fact of life and forming habits and using the chair wisely allow you to control the impact of a chair-dwelling lifestyle on your physical and mental self. The chair is a tool to be used with a purpose, a purpose of leaving as little of a metabolic imprint on your body as possible.

You can be the successful person you want to be. Instead of giving the chair-sitting energy away to maintaining a chair-sitting world, you harness the energy to do your bidding.

Here's your chance to use your time effectively. By becoming consciously aware of chair use and moving-around time, you will master your metabolism and body. You'll lessen the risk for a long list of lifestyle conditions.

What's the recipe for success? It's un-sitting your life, replacing some of your sitting time with an activity appropriate to re-setting your metabolic clock. It's more, however. It's knowing

CASE STUDY: KEVIN'S STRATEGY

For un-sitting his life Kevin originally included a standing work station for some working hours and a standing station for the evening while watching television and using an iPad. He placed a reflexology mat underfoot at these times. Kevin was seldom standing still, preferring to shift from foot to foot. He usually stood on his mat for one and a half hours per evening. Since then he's revised his program and is wearing a tracker to measure 12,000 or more steps during a day. He takes a walk each morning, bounce-steps on a mini trampoline for 15 minutes after meals, and takes breaks from sitting every hour. Kevin prefers to use a timer to time his activities.

that you are in charge, that you can change your lifestyle. You can be the successful person you want to be. Instead of giving the chair-sitting energy away to maintaining a chair-sitting world, you harness the energy to do your bidding.

It's knowing that you are in charge, that you can change your lifestyle.

The rewards? You'll know you're feeding your body the right stuff. Your body is receiving the nutrients it needs to automatically and unconsciously maintain its metabolism and other functions. You'll feel better. You'll live longer. And, as time goes by, it'll be a part of your life, not an onerous duty. Free yourself from the shackles of the chair and your mind will follow.

Consider your opportunities to move more
Much of moving more can be done in the background of your life. It could be adding more moving time during your work-day sales calls. If you then park further away from your destination and climb stairs when there's a choice, you'll have no problem meeting a 10,000-steps-a-day goal.

Create a routine
Many days include a repeated pattern of activities. Once you have considered your chances to move more, create a plan for a movement routine. Try adapting your daily office routine to add steps during breaks, take a walk during lunch, and climb stairs when possible. Use your evenings for a routine that adds more steps as well.

Make plans to move throughout the day
The reflex "diet" is all about timing. Moving throughout the day resets your metabolism and muscles, allowing you to reach your goals. The journey to work, being at work, and being at home in the evening all present opportunities to move more.

Consider your evening. Are you tempted to spend the evening sitting, tired after the day at work? Remember: the time you spend at mundane chores helps normalize your metabolism.

MOVEMENT REMINDERS

Once you have devised a more active routine for yourself, moving more will become a habit, which needs to be constantly reinforced. It needs to become a complete life change for your reflex "diet" to succeed. Reminders to remind you to move more will help you to build your habit and there are a myriad ways to do this. You can try placing an ordinary timer where you will see it to measure your efforts or a red sticker on the television set to remind you to get up during commercials. Apps on your cell phone and prompts on a computer serve as reminders as well. Then there are rewards for sticking to the program: tracking your day-to-day success or rewarding yourself for meeting your daily goal.

Spend 15 minutes cleaning the kitchen after eating and you've helped normalize blood-sugar levels. Spend 30 minutes and you've helped metabolize fats, cholesterol, and triglycerides.

It's your choice

Choose what you like to do. That way you're more likely to carry through. Try taking a walk in the morning, for example, to see what's going on in your neighborhood and perhaps visit with friends near by. In bad weather you can step in place on a mini trampoline while listening to your favorite music.

There are ways to make adding steps to your day more interesting. Try walking on a reflexology mat in the evening while you are reading or watching television. Listening to music adds to the whole experience.

If you find yourself not moving about as much as you'd like, don't be afraid to change your plans.

Change your plan if it's not working

At the end of a week, consider how much you're up and about. If you find yourself not moving about as much as you'd like, don't be afraid to change your plans.

ADD MOVEMENT TO YOUR LIFE

Whatever it is you're doing, can you add movement to your activity? Be creative. Stand and walk in place while watching television or pace while talking on the phone. If you're listening to music, reading, checking emails, or using an electronic device, use a standing station to hold your device and walk in place. Or, step in place on a mini-trampoline. Use a sit-stand desk at the office, raising your laptop or keyboard and monitor to a standing position.

Play with your children or take your dog for a long walk. Or, what about some activity, such as gardening, that you never normally find time to do? Here's your chance to add more action to your day.

Once you start, you'll find yourself looking for more steps to add to your day. A trip to the grocery store is a chance to park further away and then accumulate more steps as you walk to the front entrance. Making it fun can be even more motivating.

Make preparations

Just as you equip the kitchen before you cook, set the scene to promote the success of your reflex "diet". Think of it as "reflex-scaping", putting in place the rocking chair, having the timer handy, or buying a fitness tracker. Think ahead so that the tools are available to make it easier for you to follow your "diet". Set the scene where you spend your sitting time, to meet your goal.

Setting the scene at home

What do you do in the evening at home? Prepare everything so that you can carry out your plan. Move things into position to make moving easier and more tempting.

Setting the scene at work

Map your route so that you are taking more steps during the day: think about taking a long lunchtime walk with a coworker,

DECONSTRUCTING YOUR TIME-SAVING MEASURES

Moving more may be a matter of deconstructing the time-saving, step-saving measures you've built into your life. Is the printer conveniently located within reach of your desk chair? Could you move it further away and take more steps? You may be missing an opportunity to be getting up and moving for even a brief period of time. To give an extreme example, a man spent his evening in his recliner situated next to a beer dispenser. This meant he didn't even get his metabolism moving by walking to the fridge for a beer.

for example. Visit a colleague's office instead of emailing or calling; stand or walk around during phone calls; visit a rest room further from your office. In addition, improve your work station to accommodate easy standing or stand-sit positions.

Think about your shoes

If you're walking and standing more, you'll want your feet to be comfortable. Consider the shoes you wear. You'll want your feet to be comfortable as you add more steps to your day. Think about not wearing any shoes and going barefoot or in socks around the house. Your feet will have an opportunity to maintain their natural shape since they conform to the surfaces that surround them. Shoes enclose the foot and create uniform hard surfaces underfoot.

Keep a reflex "diet" diary

Take note of your efforts and the results. Start with measurements such as your weight and waistline or even biomarkers such as blood pressure, waistline measurements, cholesterol, or triglyceride. Keep track of the reflex techniques you apply over a particular period of time.

Reflex "diet" plan for those with mobility limits

For some people, getting up and moving about is a challenge. Foot problems, walking difficulties, recent surgery, or a disability can be an impediment. Think about how to deal with this. Benefits can be obtained through rocking in a rocking chair, using an electric foot vibrator, or activities such as hand crafts or reflexology self-applied techniques.

ACTIVE TELEVISION TIME

As one researcher noted, the problem with television-viewing isn't watching television as such, but that the "default" position for television-watching is sitting. Keep in mind what another researcher said: if television-watching time were converted to active time, many health problems could be avoided. The solution is to add movement to your television-watching time. Why not create a strategy to enhance your sitting time while you watch television: read, knit, or pursue a hobby, use a rocking chair, an electric foot roller or a vibrating electric foot platform. Apply self-hand or foot reflexology techniques too. Try standing and walking in place at every television commercial.

Be up and about as you watch television. An at-home standing station within view of the television creates a usable surface for holding your computer device (video gaming, laptop, iPad, tablet, iPod), phone, book, or hobby materials. Enhance your efforts by placing a reflexology mat underfoot.

Position your exercise equipment so that it faces the television (such as a treadmill equipped with a holding stand). This provides an opportunity to read, use your laptop, or other device while you are exercising. Harvard researcher Dr. Frank Hu watches television from his treadmill. Free-standing exercises, weight-lifting, or other exercise activities are good to try as well. Walk on a reflexology mat, practice tai chi, yoga, or Pilates.

CASE STUDY: BARBARA'S STRATEGY

When Barbara's sitting at the computer during the day, her feet rest on a vibrating foot platform. She takes two-minute breaks from sitting every 15 or 20 minutes, timed by the foot platform turning itself off. A two-minute break is timed by noting 200 steps on the wearable fitness tracker. She walks on a reflexology mat for 15 minutes after meals, timed by watching the clock.

In the evening, the television may be on while she is walking on a reflexology mat after dinner and, when seated in a rocking chair, an electric foot roller or vibrating foot platform is underfoot. She's usually reading and frequently applies hands-on foot and hand reflexology. Two-minute breaks continue through the evening. Timing two hours more throughout the day is done by noting steps on the wearable fitness tracker. By the end of the day, she's taken 12,000 to 14,000 steps as measured on the tracker. She works out following hip flexor exercises.

Design a healthier, happier you

Do you have a health concern? Are you happy with how it's going or frustrated with your lack of progress? Are you worried about a health condition that runs in your family? Is longevity one of your key goals? Perhaps your interest is preventive, maintaining quality of life and doing what you can to stay healthy, both mentally and physically.

To achieve your goal, you'll want to define it. First, let's consider key motivations you might have for using the reflex "diet": I want to be slimmer; I want a "better me"; I want to feel and look good; I want to have more energy. What is it you want? Any of the above is possible with a focused effort using the reflex "diet". To work toward your goal, make your efforts objective and measurable. When you see the effects of what you've done, it provides motivation to go further.

CASE STUDY: THE "FAT GENE"

Take, for example, one young woman who states that she's got the "fat gene". She bases this on the evidence of weight problems in the family and all her unsuccessful efforts to lose weight. Maybe she's really inherited the "sitting-too-much gene".

There is what researcher Dr. David Levine considers to be a genetic predisposition to sit too much. but that's not the whole story. The woman applied the reflex "diet" principles, gradually adding more steps per day as measured by a fitness tracker, taking more steps around the office, and parking on a different level. She's been able to measure her progress in weight lost as well as in lost inches.

Timing your movement is critical. You need to know you're up and moving frequently enough to know you're making a difference. Use a timer, wearable fitness tracer, or pedometer to measure your effort. Track your efforts over time by keeping a reflex diary or using the technology linking wearable fitness tracker to a smartphone or computer. You'll know what your performance is. Now you'll be able to build a profile and have an indicator of your performance over time.

You'll know how often you're meeting your performance goal and such information will serve as motivation. One client noted that if it's 10 o'clock at night and he hasn't reached his 10,000 steps, he starts stepping in place to achieve his goals. Then there's another client who takes steps as he waits for his glass to be filled by the water dispenser in the refrigerator door.

Moving about more needs to become a habit for your reflex "diet" to succeed.

In essence, what you are aiming for and how you achieve it becomes a game when the necessity, which is moving around more, becomes fun. If you follow the reflex "diet" but it feels like a chore, it's a lot harder to achieve your goals.

Think about creating a goal that you are willing and able to commit to. Then think about your choices: basic maintenance, weight improvement, improving metabolic indicators; lessening risk for lifestyle conditions, musculoskeletal concerns, cognitive decline, and aging better. You can then commit to that goal with specifics. How much change do you want to see, for example, in your blood pressure?

A client noted that if it's 10 o'clock at night and he hasn't reached his 10,000 steps, he starts stepping in place to achieve his goals.

Think you may have low start-up energy?

Here's a test. Have you dropped something on the floor and considered whether or not to pick it up because you don't have enough energy to do it? If so, you have very low start-up energy.

➥ First, just get started. If you can take that first step, it's easier to take the next one. Consider taking small steps, gradually building up to more and more reflex activities.

➥ Convince yourself to do a little and then a little more. You can make a difference in as little as two minutes.

➥ Imagine a positive result for yourself. And, when you do achieve it, seize on it to motivate further activity.

How do you grab more energy?

Tired after your day at work? Even though you might think that you need to relax and take things easy, you can actually grab more energy when you're tired by getting moving again.

CASE STUDY: EFFECTS ON TYPE-TWO DIABETES

A clerk who was working at a big box store was diagnosed with type-two diabetes. He changed his diet, started exercising daily, and continued his job with its pedometer-verified 10,000 steps a day. Six months later, testing showed he was no longer diabetic and today he continues his diet, daily exercise, and job.

GETTING STARTED ON YOUR "DIET"

Is it difficult to get started or engaged in getting more active and succeeding in your "diet"? Do you find yourself moving less rather than more? Are you seeing any results? Consider:

→ It's important to carry out your "diet" in your own way, so that it works for you. Choose the up-and-about schedule and activity that you like and will want to do. If you like it, you'll do it.

→ Customize your reflex strategy and fit it into your life seamlessly. Experiment and see what works for you.

→ Do you struggle to get out of your chair to stand and walk about during the evenings? You may feel tired at the end of the work day and if you stand and walk all day, you may feel you can't stand any more. This is understandable. You need a well-deserved rest, but the danger is you'll remain stationary for hours at a time. However, whatever your thoughts, your body has its own reflex schedule and it needs to be up and moving.

→ Find a starting point. Can you get out of your chair for five minutes whenever television programs change?

→ What will motivate you to help your body? One person was motivated by the desire to see his grandchildren grow up.

→ Don't be a perfectionist. If you fall off the wagon and stop your "diet", start it up again and you'll soon see results once more.

→ Don't judge yourself harshly. Maybe you haven't yet found the right combination of factors to get you going. Take a break and re-evaluate your progress. Perhaps get support by enlisting a friend to encourage you and even join you in your regime.

→ When you have achieved your goal, reward yourself. Give yourself a treat. Tell your friends about your accomplishments and get their feedback.

Low-intensity physical activity (walking, standing, and activities done while walking and standing) has been shown to reduce fatigue. "Although it seems inconsistent, walking can actually energize tired bodies. ... a University of Georgia study found that low-intensity exercise, like walking, can increase your energy level by 20% and decrease fatigue by 65%."

Part two

REFLEX TECHNIQUES

5 Sitting smart

There are a variety of active sitting techniques that are simple yet provide benefits that counteract the negatives associated with sitting.

As you're doing more than one thing at a time, you're stacking activities, and perhaps doing things that will improve both your body and mind at the same time. Rocking, for example, causes more blood to be sent to the heart and brain, therefore improving your blood pressure, your brain power, and your mood.

Imagine a device you could sit in that enhances your sitting time, eating up twice the calories as sitting in a regular chair. It's known as a rocking chair.

Whatever kind of chair you use, when you sit, sit with a purpose. Think about how long you sit uninterrupted for and make every moment count. Become a rocker and strategize your rocking. Chairs that rock at the office, in the dining room, or living room can become your mini-gym, working the postural muscles of your feet and legs.

But there's more. Very important postural muscles can be activated while you are sitting still. Machines that vibrate, roll, or bathe the feet have been shown to reverse, eliminate, or improve some of the negative effects of sitting on the cardiovascular system. Think of a workout going on under your feet as you are sitting down.

Sitting: the recipe for success

How much sitting is too much? Good question. There is a recipe for success that meets the needs of our inner cave-dweller. The best answer is if you've sat for an hour, you've sat for too long. All sorts of metabolic processes start to shut down after an hour of sitting. So a five-minute break is suggested every hour, but

THINK ABOUT YOUR METABOLIC RATE

→ Lying down (but not asleep) results in the lowest metabolic rate.

→ Time spent watching television results in the lowest metabolic rate of all seated activities. Even for those who exercise regularly or who work at a standing/walking job during the day, time spent watching television in the evening has negative consequences.

→ Thirty minutes of exercise is negated by one hour of sitting, according to one study, and three hours of sitting by another.

it also depends on your goals. A two-minute break in sitting is suggested every 20 minutes if you have concerns about blood sugar, blood pressure, or musculoskeletal aches and pains.

What does an hour of sitting mean to the inner "you"? Many people have become educated to the caloric and other consequences of eating a particular food. Think chocolate eclair versus garden salad. Here we consider the metabolic consequences of sitting.

The best chair is the one you leave often.

Killer chairs

Lurking there, in plain sight, and in every corner of our indoor and outdoor worlds – it's the killer chair. Yes, it's a mandatory, 90-degree world for our bodies as we sit in the conventionally accepted mini-environment. And, as scientists are now telling us, it's a piece of furniture that, over time, will kill us.

Maximize your chair use

The chair can help create an environment that allows more movement, contributing to "motion promotion", encouraging "a variety of postures and movements throughout our day to feel our best, and integrating more movement throughout our days instead of merely activity sandwiched into a period of exercise." The best chair is the one you leave often, but given that we have to use them sometimes, what are the best options? Not all chairs are created equal.

THE EXERCISE-BALL CHAIR

Maintaining balance as one sits on an exercise ball, a large inflatable plastic ball to improve core muscles and balance, requires minute adjustments and engages the postural muscles. Sitting on a ball burns 4 more calories an hour than sitting in a chair, or about 30 extra calories in a work day. Anne Spalding and Linda Kelly observe what exercise-ball seating can provide for school children. "Some of the rewards for using exercise balls in the classroom are simply this: happy, focused, and productive kids ... Many kids and adults who have a great deal of trouble sitting still are given the chance on the ball to move in an appropriate way and get some exercise while situated in what many people and educators may have formerly seen as a sedentary environment."

→ A chair that allows the feet to rest on the floor is good. It allows some pressure to be applied to the feet.

→ The recliner is the "high heel" of chairs. Lying back in a recliner places the body in a position of lying down, creating a reduced metabolic demand. Good recliner use is when the recliner is upright, with your feet on the floor or while rocking.

→ An ottoman or stool, which elevates the feet, has impact on the metabolism similar to lying back in a recliner.

→ An exercise-ball chair is a good alternative because it allows the body to shift around and burn up more calories.

→ A chair that allows a rocking motion provides an opportunity to flex your leg muscles as you rock, with the good things that ensue. Rocking features are included with some office chairs, recliners, and dining-room chairs.

Rocking-chair medicine

While most of us call it a "rocking chair" some researchers have a different take. Some refer to it as "therapy" or even a "medical device". Whatever its name, rocking creates improvements in physical and mental wellbeing.

RESEARCH ON ROCKING-CHAIR THERAPY

Rocking-chair therapy is the term used by Dr. Nancy Watson of the University of Rochester, New York, following her research findings as having physical and emotional benefits for nursing-home residents, especially those with Alzheimer's. It is also a term used by those who work with ADHD children.

Dr. Heinrich Addleheim of the Kinetic Therapy Clinic in Berlin, Germany, says, "it's not just a piece of furniture; it's a remarkable medical device. ... We've seen cases of patients recuperating from heart attack and stroke – without any trace of permanent damage – simply because they used a rocking chair while they were recovering. I've seen people bedridden with arthritis who were up and around inside a week after regular use of rocking chair."

HOW SITTING/ROCKING IMPACTS BLOOD PRESSURE

One study showed that 20 minutes of quiet sitting lowered blood pressure for half the women in the study and raised it for the other half. Another study showed that 30 minutes of rocking normalized low blood pressure.

Rocking in a rocking chair puts into action postural muscles of the calves with benefits including: causing twice the calories of quiet sitting to be expended, normalizing blood pressure, sending more blood to the brain, improving balance and walking mechanisms, mood, and emotions, as well as reducing pain. Rocking is seen as a mild form of exercise for the elderly or for those with difficulties walking.

Rocking-chair reflex actions
Rocking initiates reflex actions prompted by movement of the postural muscles of the calves, leading to improvements

in blood pressure, balance, blood to the brain, and endorphin release. The rocking chair becomes therapy as rocking puts into action the calf muscles. Rocking with toes pointed engages postural muscles and some of the activities of standing or walking are mimicked. As calf muscles contract and relax, their veins compress and decompress, pumping blood from the extremities and helping it return to the brain and heart. The net result is a normalizing of blood pressure and a brain with more blood available.

Brain food by rocking

Blood means life for the brain, with 20% of the blood pumped by the heart traveling to the brain, carrying glucose used for energy. Rocking in a rocking chair contributes to cerebral profusion, the availability of blood to the brain. This is what one researcher found when examining why rocking benefitted residents of a dementia unit. Rocking for 70 minutes accumulated throughout the day had an impact noticed by staff members and family alike of a ward for dementia residents. Rocking reduced pain medication requests, anxiety, depression, and agitation. Those who rocked the most saw improvements in balance and mobility.

Rocking and balance and mobility

The rocking motion stimulates the vestibular apparatus of the inner ears, important for informing the body about its position, contributing to information used to create settings appropriate to sitting or standing. It helps determine blood-pressure levels, increasing with the demands of standing and walking while decreasing with sitting.

The vestibular apparatus is tied to maintaining the balance important to walking abilities, helping explain the improvements noted above. In one study significant improvements in mobility-related activities such as balance, walking speed, and rising out of a chair more easily were seen by elderly women who rocked twice a day for 15 minutes compared to women who didn't.

Moreover, researchers note that the program was easily implemented, with rocking participants becoming motivated and continuing after the study. "This is a promising alternative exercise method for maintaining physical activity and it leads to improvements in physical performance."

Calorie-counting and rocking

Perhaps some explanation for the benefits of rocking lie in the additional expenditure of calories. Rocking in a rocking chair is reported to double the number of calories expended by the body as compared to sitting quietly – 150 calories per hour as compared to 71 to 84, depending on the person's weight.

Expending more calories through increased activity is seen by Dr. James Levine to create improvements in metabolism. His theory involves moving about for two additional hours a day. However, calories expended when using a rocking chair would benefit those who have difficulty moving. The elderly who engaged in activities requiring 1,000 additional calories a day through daily activities saw a significantly reduced incidence of dementia. Rocking would contribute to the expenditure of calories.

Rocking in a rocking chair is reported to double the number of calories consumed as compared to sitting quietly.

Endorphin release and rocking

Endorphin release, similar to a runner's high, may help explain why less pain medication was requested by the elderly who rocked.

Who benefits from "rocking-chair medicine"?

Research shows the benefits of rocking-chair use for the elderly, reducing pain, anxiety, depression, and agitation as well as improving balance and mobility, especially important for nursing-home residents and those with Alzheimer's.

ADHD children: The comforting motion of a rocking chair helps calm ADHD children. They are able to move as they read, listen, and learn, which seems to improve their concentration and focus. The net result is a calmer child, who retains more

RESEARCH ON DEMENTIA

Widespread interest in the therapeutic benefits of rocking chairs for the elderly resulted from a 1998 study by researcher Dr. Nancy Watson from the University of Rochester School of Nursing. She studied rocking-chair use by nursing-home residents with dementia. "Rocking immediately calmed the residents down and, over six weeks, lessened crying or expressions of anxiety with tension and depression dropping in 11." She found that study participants who rocked 101 minutes per day on average – throughout the day, not necessarily consecutively – also showed reductions in pain medication related to the amount of rocking. The more rocking, the greater the reduction. Significant improvements in balance were found by those who liked rocking and wanted to continue it at the end of the study.

information and participates better. Rocking-chair use for children is growing in schools, child-care centers, and homes.

Infants: Being rocked in a rocking chair is soothing and comforting for babies. For infants being rocked, the rhythmic motion also provides stimulation to the vestibular apparatus of the ears, the balance center, promoting the baby's ability to be alert and attentive as well as helping with the development of balance mechanisms.

Dementia sufferers: See box above.

The workout under your feet

Self-applied hand and foot reflexology while you are sitting will give you a benefical workout under your feet.

Ball-rolling

Rolling a tennis ball on the sole of the foot relaxes the hamstring muscles of the legs that may have tightened during prolonged

The Rocking Chair Project charity provides mothers with rocking chairs to aid development during the crucial early months of an infant's life.

sitting, impeding a full range of motion and an efficient gait. You can place a tennis ball under your office desk or in front of your easy chair. But do remember to tuck it away so that it won't trip you when you stand up.

Foot-entertainment units

There are many types of foot-entertainment units available to help not just your feet feel better but have an impact on reflex activity and physiological measures. The feet have multi-sensory responsibilities, including not only the perception of pressure, stretch, and movement but also heat and cold. Your feet are teeming with sensors trying to figure out what's going on. Think of it as entertaining your feet while benefitting your health.

Your feet are teeming with sensors trying to figure out what's going on.

Foot-stimulating electric machines that vibrate, roll, or bathe the feet have been shown to impact one measure of sitting too much, reduced heart-rate variability.

Heart-rate variability, the interval between heart beats, is seen to be healthier if it varies. Heart-rate variability is seen as an indicator of the ability to adapt to stress and a measure of the state of the autonomic nervous system, which controls functions of the heart, breathing, the digestive system, and the endocrine glands. "Decreased heart rate variability is associated with a higher risk of mortality" and "increased risk of CV (cardiovascular) disease, type-two diabetes and insulin resistance", according to prolonged sitting researchers at Pennington Biomedical Research Center.

Vibrating foot platform

The use of a vibrating foot platform completely reversed the effects of quiet sitting on the cardiovascular system. Blood pressure and heart-rate variability were normalized. For many of us, sitting is a relaxing activity with blood pressure and cardiac stress falling. But this is not so for everyone. For half of the participants of one study, sitting had a profound effect on the cardiovascular system. Blood pressure and other measures

RESEARCH ON FIDGETING

Fidgeting is your body's way of telling you that it wants to move, but it's also a category of seated activity. Fidgeting while sitting may be why computer use, reading, knitting, or driving are less impactful on the metabolism.

Research by Dr. James Levine of the Mayo Clinic showed that those who sit motionless burn 80 calories an hour while those who fidget while sitting burn 118 calories per hour. In his research, "Activities (performed by participants that resulted in increased calorie expenditure) tended to be consistent between subjects and included hand and foot tapping and arm and leg swinging. Most subjects did not move their trunks noticeably; eight read magazines and three performed hair-grooming gestures and computer work."

Keep in mind that there is still an adverse impact to sitting while engaged in another activity too. A 113% increased risk of heart attack or stroke was seen in men who spend more than four hours a day of non-work-related screen time (TV-viewing, surfing the internet or playing video games) compared to those who spent less than two hours a day.

of cardiovascular stress acted abnormally and went up instead of down. The reason? The cardiovascular system adjusts as we sit, compensating for the lack of movement by leg muscles. Muscle tone helps veins in the legs return blood to the heart from the extremities. For these participants, sitting was a cardiovascular stress as their hearts worked harder to maintain blood pressure while sitting because of a hypothesized lack of muscle tone in the legs.

Fidgeting is your body's way of telling you that it wants to move.

RESEARCH ON FOOT-BATHING

Japanese researchers found that a 10-minute foot bath created physiological changes beneficial to health. A foot bath with bubbles and vibration in water at 105° created significant changes in heart-rate variability as measured by an ECG, demonstrating change in autonomic response and "indicating a shift to increased parasympathetic and decreased sympathetic activity".

Also found were "significant increases in white blood cell (WBC) count and natural killer (NK) cell cytotoxicity, suggesting an improved immune status".

The use of a vibrating foot platform completely reversed the effects of quiet sitting on the cardiovascular system as measured by blood pressure and heart-rate variability for all study participants, according to researcher Dr. Guruprasad Madhavan of the State University of New York, Binghamton.

Why would this be? The vibrating foot platform is thought to create the same frequency on the sole of the foot as the sensations perceived by receptors on the soles of the feet as one stands and walks. These receptors communicate with the postural muscles, helping to set the tone for muscles as well as the activity of the inner "you".

Electric foot roller

The 20-minute use of an electric foot roller applied to the heart reflex area (the ball of the left foot, below the big toe) significantly changed heart-rate variability. The researchers speculated that improved circulation of blood from feet to heart creates a situation where "there will be more variation in the heart rate and become more chaotic". As discussed earlier, this is a good thing.

SUMMARY OF THE BENEFITS OF SITTING SMART

Rocking chair

➥Causes twice the calories of quiet sitting to be expended

➥Normalizes blood pressure

➥Sends more blood to the brain

➥Improves balance and walking mechanisms

➥Improves mood and emotions

➥Reduces pain

➥Introduces a mild form of exercise for the elderly or for those with difficulties walking

Ball-rolling

➥Relaxes some muscles tightened during prolonged sitting

Vibrating foot platform

➥Reverses effects of quiet sitting on blood pressure and heart-rate variability

Electric foot roller

➥Significant change in heart-rate variability

6 Take a break

Taking two-minute breaks in sitting normalizes metabolism for our inner cave-dweller thrown into disarray by sitting too much. A 90-second break re-sets the metabolism, while a two-minute break re-sets the metabolism and muscles.

This means that taking breaks in sitting could be the answer for reaching your body-behavior goals: re-setting your metabolism, increasing calorie consumption, re-shaping your body's appearance, creating a smaller waistline, lowering blood pressure, as well as reducing risk for falls and injury, musculoskeletal discomfort, risk for diabetes, and risk for gait problems later in life. Improved is performance at work, learning, and behavior for children at school and in sports performance.

Taking breaks in sitting could be the answer for reaching your body behavior goals.

What happens when you don't take breaks? A computer engineer disabled the signal installed by his company to remind him to take a break. He is normally confined to his chair concentrating, which works fine for the initial four hours of the work day. However, he reports that he doesn't get much done for the second half of the day since he's "wiped out". Then there's the client who got up faithfully at 5am to attend a spin class, then went home and sat in her office chair for four-hour spells of concentrated work. She's unable to meet her weight-loss goal. Neither was satisfied with how their bodies were working – perhaps explained by the lack of breaks in sitting being taken.

Barbara continued searching for the best office chair to stave off neck pain, but found that the chair itself was not the problem. Rather, taking breaks in sitting ended her search.

How frequently are breaks in sitting needed? And, what should you do while you are taking a break? Good questions and the answer is up to you. What are your goals? What is practical for you to do? Do you have physical limitations?

How often should you take a break in sitting?

Best practice is to take a break in sitting of two minutes every 20, involving moving about or walking in place. This creates more contractions of the postural muscles and patterns of pressure to the feet than standing. Benefits include normalization of the musculoskeletal system, blood-sugar level, and the cardiovascular system. However, taking a standing break

RESEARCH ON TAKING BREAKS

Research finds those who take the most breaks benefit the most. Researcher Dr. Genevieve Healy of the University of Queensland, Australia, found that those who take the most breaks during the day had better biomarkers for metabolism and a lessened risk for heart disease and diabetes. "Even one minute of standing (while taking a break in sitting) made a difference in various indicators of risk for heart disease, metabolic diseases such as diabetes, and inflammatory processes that can play a role in atherosclerosis (blocked [hardening of the] arteries)."

In a study published in the *European Heart Journal*, Healy et al. found that the more breaks from sitting taken by an individual, the less the impact of sitting on both the waistline and indicators of heart health.

for as little as a minute can be beneficial. If you've sat for an hour, you've sat too long. This is one thing on which researchers can all agree. While there is no definitive answer to the question "how often should breaks in sitting be taken", various researchers have documented the benefits of taking breaks at set intervals.

If you've sat an hour, you've sat too long.

What taking breaks can do for you
➥One-minute breaks
Cancer prevention: One-minute breaks can lower biomarkers associated with cancer risk. Researcher Dr. Nevill Owen of Australia notes, "In our studies, we've measured waist circumference, insulin resistance and inflammation – indicators of cancer risk common to many physical activity-cancer studies. We found that even breaks as short as one minute can lower these biomarkers."

➥Ninety-second breaks
According to researcher Dr. James Levine, "... within 90 seconds of standing up, the muscular and cellular systems that process blood sugar, triglycerides, and cholesterol – which are mediated by insulin – are activated." If you've sat an hour, "the cellular mechanisms involved in the maintenance of your body and health are shutting down."

➥Five-minute break every hour
Blood flow: a five-minute break every hour improves blood flow and relieves musculoskeletal discomfort. Sitting for one hour impaired the functioning of the main artery of the leg by 50% due to lack of blood flow. Walking for five minutes every hour returned the function of the artery to normal, according to researchers at the University of Indiana.

Musculoskeletal discomfort: Several studies showed effectiveness in relieving musculoskeletal discomfort with a five-minute break every hour (aside from typical on-the-job mid-morning, mid-afternoon, and lunch breaks).

➥Two-minute break every 20 minutes
Blood pressure: Both systolic and diastolic blood pressure were

significantly lowered (by three points each) when a group of study participants took two-minute breaks from sitting every 20 minutes, compared to when they sat completely uninterrupted for seven hours.

Insulin/glucose metabolism/cardiovascular risk: Higher glucose levels after eating are a risk factor for cardiovascular disease. When overweight/obese adults took two-minute breaks every 20 minutes over a five-hour period following a meal, glucose and insulin levels were lower compared to sitting for five hours after a meal. Researchers note: "This may improve glucose metabolism and potentially be an important public health and clinical intervention strategy for reducing cardiovascular risk."

Figure-shaping, gait, sports performance: musculoskeletal goals: Taking a two- or three-minute break every 20 or 30 minutes is suggested to prevent the long-term impact on the lower back, hips and pelvis by muscles tightened by sitting too much, the hip flexors. The end result is an unstable base for walking, playing sports, and day-to-day activities. Impacted as well is the shape of the body, with a big behind and pot belly forming. At risk later in life is the ability to walk and concerns about falls. At risk over years are performance and injury playing sports or just moving through the day. Hip flexors tighten during prolonged sitting, impeding a full range of

IS 20 MINUTES A MAGIC NUMBER?

Engage in physical activity every 20 minutes and you'll live healthier and for longer. Dan Buettner, author of *The Blue Zones Solution: Eating and Living Like the World's Healthiest People*, found cultures around the world whose residents live the healthiest and longest are "nudged into physical activity (such as housework, yard work, kitchen work with no mechanized appliances) every 20 minutes, my team estimates. This activity not only burned 500 to 1,000 calories a day; it also kept their metabolisms humming at a high rate."

motion and an efficient gait. Getting up and moving every 20 to 30 minutes for two to three minutes will relax these muscles.

Musculoskeletal discomfort: Taking a microbreak of 30 seconds every 20 minutes helped computer workers who reported frequent or long-term neck, shoulder, wrist, and/or finger discomfort. Discomfort was reduced while there was "no evidence of a detrimental effect on worker productivity" in one Dutch study. Other studies showed effectiveness at relieving musculoskeletal discomfort with a five-minute break every hour (aside from mid-morning, mid-afternoon, and lunch breaks) or four breaks an hour (three 30-second micro-breaks and a three-minute break). Stretching and/or walking away from the work station were advocated.

Learning: Moving about every 20 minutes enhances the learning experience for children and improves student behavior. Brain researcher Eric Jensen "recommends that students and adults need to move approximately every 20 minutes. ... Movement improves brain development, increases nerve connections, and solidifies learning. These energizers wake up learners, increase their energy levels, improve their information storage and retrieval to help them feel good. A very short break or energizer increases arousal but longer breaks allow the learner to be aroused and then come back to a more sustainable level of energy."

⮕ **Break every 30 minutes**
Calories: Taking a break in sitting eats up more calories. Taking a walking break for one minute every half an hour results in the expenditure of an additional 24 calories over an eight-hour period; a two-minute break results in 59 extra calories expended and a five-minute break results in 132 additional calories expended, as reported in research by Dr. Ann Swartz of the University of Wisconsin at Milwaukee. Not much, you might think, but remember: researchers studied the impact of how sedentary jobs impact weight. Using data accumulated since 1970, they found the resulting lessened expenditure of calories

Taking a break in sitting eats up more calories.

to be 100 calories a day – enough to account for a significant portion of the increase in weight gain experienced by women and men in the US over the intervening years.

➥ 15-minute break after eating

Blood-sugar level: Ever heard you should take a walk after a heavy meal? Well, it turns out to be good advice. A 24% reduction in glucose levels resulted when middle-aged women engaged in 15 or 40 minutes of light-intensity physical activity (activities of daily living: cooking, washing dishes, ironing, and other routine domestic or occupational tasks done while standing or walking). Glucose levels raised by a carbohydrate-rich meal were normalized. Lowered were high blood-sugar levels that increase the risk of diabetes. This was in comparison to those who sat for two hours after a carbohydrate-rich meal, who, as a result, researchers stated "had a clinically significant increase in metabolic risk".

> *Ever heard you should take a walk after a heavy meal? Well, it turns out to be good advice.*

➥ Break taken while stepping in place during television commercial breaks

Standing up and stepping in place during commercial breaks while television-viewing adds steps to one's day – as much as 3,000 steps over 90-minutes. "The standard half-hour TV show contains 8–12 minutes of commercials. Thus, for the average person who watches 2.6 hours/day of television there are approximately 40–60 minutes of commercials," according to researcher graduate student Jeremy Adam Steeves of the University of Tennessee. The 58 participants in his study did not lose weight during the three weeks of study.

Calories: Watching television for an hour while stepping in place during the commercials resulted in 148 calories being burnt. Reclining or seated television-viewing expended 81 and 79 calories respectively, while one hour of commercial stepping resulted in an average of about 25 minutes of physical activity and 2,000 steps.

TAKING BREAKS FROM SITTING

CALORIES	
1-, 2-, 5-minute break every ½ hour	Results in an expenditure of an extra 24, 59, 132 calories in an 8-hour day

CANCER PREVENTIVE	
1–2-minute breaks	Can lower cancer risk biomarkers (waist circumference, insulin resistance, inflammation)

CARDIOVASCULAR DISEASE	
1–2-minute breaks	Can lower inflammation, a biomarker risk for cardiovascular disease

INSULIN/GLUCOSE METABOLISM/CARDIOVASCULAR DISEASE	
A 2-minute break every 20 minutes following a meal	Lowers glucose and insulin levels, improving glucose metabolism, and reducing cardiovascular risk

METABOLIC SYNDROME	
1-minute standing breaks, with those taking the most breaks making most difference	Makes a difference in indicators for risk of heart disease, metabolic disease (diabetes), and inflammatory processes (atherosclerosis)

PAIN/PROFICIENCY (MUSCULOSKELETAL)	
2-minute breaks every 20 minutes	Relieves muscle, ligament, and spine stress, leg venous system: decreasing discomfort/improved mobility proficiency, figure-shaping, sports performance

SUMMARY OF THE BENEFITS OF TAKING BREAKS

The body has a reflex effect, an automatic, unconscious response to taking breaks in sitting. Benefits of taking breaks are:

→ Re-sets metabolic mechanisms (cholesterol, triglycerides, waistline, blood pressure, insulin resistance, and blood glucose)
→ Re-sets the musculoskeletal system to prevent: lack of proficiency in walking (especially later in life) and moving-about activities such as sports; changes in physical appearance (big behind and pot belly)
→ Lessens musculoskeletal discomfort
→ Increases calorie expenditure
→ Creates a smaller waistline
→ Provides more blood to the brain and heart
→ Improves biomarkers for cancer and cardiovascular risk
→ Improves learning and behavior in children
→ Improves performance in adults

7 Steps to sharpen your reflexes

You've heard about sharpening your reflexes and that it's a good thing, but you probably never thought that each step you take does just that. To make your reflexes work for you, focus on how your time and effort are being spent, on the rewards you gain from what you're doing, and on the activities that have a value for you.

Here we present the value of the various techniques that work on your reflexes (a vital part of the reflex "diet"). You can decide from the menu of possibilities which one suits you best.

Standing and walking activities automatically and unconsciously feed your body the right "nutrition": the standing, walking, and moving "nutrients" it needs to maintain your body. These ingredients are free: just you and your decision to commit your time to saving yourself from the risks of chair-living. The automatic and unconscious reflexive response to sitting for any length of time creates problems. Another way of looking at it is that the reflexes are merely responding to the situation at hand (not moving for a length of time), a reflexive response of metabolic and other settings appropriate to sitting results. Unfortunately, the responses are not the best thing for us and our health.

To consider why prolonged sitting creates problems, think about the body's response to exercise. As research has shown, exercise has an effect on the workings of the body and is measured by its "dose": duration, intensity, and frequency. A workout of 30 minutes of moderate or high physical activity practiced five days a week creates healthful effects.

Next, think about the fact that your body and its reflexes are at work 24 hours a day and seven days a week. The activities of our days and nights constitute our body's daily workout. Measured by "dose", it is the duration, intensity, and frequency of our minute-by-minute, hour-by-hour, day-by-day activities that create the reflex responses that define our health and wellness.

During 16 hours of a typical day in modern-day life, a major activity, sitting, has such little intensity of effort that it is considered to be "inactivity". When practiced with duration and frequency, daily for nine hours, negative health consequences result.

Some standing and walking activities have more value than others.

While it is true that standing or walking has more value than sitting, some standing and walking activities have more value than others. More energy is expended and calories burnt as well as creating better metabolic biomarkers if you stand or walk, but standing or walking that includes an activity as well has even more value.

Taking steps

Pay attention to what you do as you move throughout the day. By substituting some of your sitting time with some moving-around time, you'll be helping to reduce your risk for obesity and metabolic dysfunction.

Standing and walking around your home or workplace is a form of low-intensity physical activity. The low-intensity activity of maintaining posture as you stand and walk happens via the actions of muscles specific to the task: postural muscles. Pressure, perceived by sensors in the feet, provides information as well. These muscles and pressure sensors perform unconscious, reflexive, actions for the purpose of keeping us upright, countering gravity, as you walk and stand. The body becomes active, with metabolism being mobilized, calorie-burning increased, and more.

Cleaning house? Be mindful of the "nutrients" you're creating for yourself.

Mundane activities as we move through the day, such as pacing while on the phone or cleaning the house, are considered light-intensity physical activities, but, in fact, they burn more than 90% of calories for those who do not exercise. This shows that such activities may be far more important to a healthy lifestyle than what we think of as "exercise" (moderate- or vigorous-intensity physical activity). As noted by author John Cloud, "Many obesity researchers now believe that very frequent, low-level physical activity – the kind humans did for tens of thousands of years before the leaf blower was invented – may actually work better for us than the occasional bouts of exercise you get as a gym rat."

Moderate- or high-intensity physical activity benefits a mechanism of the body, one different from that impacted by the light-intensity physical activity of standing and walking. For this reason, even if you exercise, the reflex actions prompted by standing and walking need a workout as well. You're ahead of those who don't exercise and sit too much, but the benefits of 30 minutes of exercise disappear with three hours of sitting, according to one researcher, and one hour according to another.

THE EFFECTS OF CUTTING BACK STEPS

One study asked active walkers to cut back on the number of steps they took each day from about 10,000 steps to 1,350 steps. They used elevators instead of stairs or drove to work. "By the end of the two weeks, all of them had became worse at metabolizing sugars and fats. Their distribution of body fat had also altered – they had become fatter around the middle. Such changes are among the first steps on the road to diabetes."

The effects of taking steps
Metabolism
Metabolism changes with activities of daily living, according to researcher Sarah M. Camhi and colleagues at Pennington Biomedical Research Center in Baton Rouge, Louisiana. Her research found that every 30 minutes or 1,000 steps taken during lifestyle activities:

➟ Lowers the risk of elevated waist circumference by 16% for every 1,000 steps or 14% for every 30 minutes.
➟ Reduces the risk of low HDL (good cholesterol) by 12% for every 1,000 steps or 11% for every 30 minutes.
➟ Lowers the risk of elevated triglycerides by 15%.
➟ Lessens the odds of having metabolic syndrome by 13%.

Alzheimer's
Among the elderly, "... activities like cooking, washing the dishes, playing cards and even moving a wheelchair with a person's arms were beneficial", created a "protective benefit" leading to reduced cognitive decline. According to Dr. Aron S. Buchman's research among participants averaging 82 years old, those who are the least physically active are 2.3 times more likely to develop Alzheimer's.

Cancer preventive
Light-intensity physical activity is significantly associated with a reduced risk of breast cancer and may have a protective effect for breast-cancer risk. Sitting time may independently contribute to breast-cancer risk. This is according to researchers who collected information about sitting and moving habits and analyzed data about biomarkers for cancer risk.

Cardiovascular disease and longevity
Being physically active around the home cut the risk of heart attack and stroke as well as improved longevity for those over the age of 60. Swedish researchers found a 27% lower risk of cardiovascular disease and 30% lower risk of death in those who engaged in a high level of physical activities around the home "... including doing home repairs, cutting the lawn or hedge, car

maintenance, going hunting or fishing, cycling, and gathering mushrooms or berries". Those who also took exercise had the lowest risk.

Taking steps around the home or office

Cleaning the home, doing gardening, or straightening up the office may be a chore, but there's more going on than meets the eye. What's the value? Such activity improves metabolism and biomarkers associated with it. The biomarkers are important to risks for stroke, heart disease, as well as for Alzheimer's, cancer, and longevity. Associated as well is maintenance of weight. Research has found that overweight individuals spend less time per day on such activities.

Counting steps

Considering the total number of steps taken throughout the day is one way of measuring light-intensity physical activity. Taking steps has been shown to make a difference in weight gain, blood pressure, waistline measurement, and longevity as well as metabolic fat and sugar levels.

USING FITNESS TRACKERS TO COUNT STEPS

Use a pedometer, a smartphone app, wearable technology such as a FitBit or VivoFit to keep track of your footsteps during the day. Choose the one that suits your purposes best. Using a pedometer can also provide an incentive to take steps. Low-activity, overweight women were, more significantly, more successful at being physically active when they aimed at taking 10,000 steps a day measured by pedometer than women who tried to do 30 minutes a day of exercise.

Women who were asked to walk 10,000 steps a day using a pedometer were more likely to be physically active over a 12-week period than those who were asked to exercise for 30 minutes a day.

A sedentary person takes 3,000 steps a day. A desk-bound person (man or woman) takes 5,000 to 6,000 steps a day. Under 5,000 steps per day is considered a "sedentary" lifestyle.

⇀If you take 2,000 additional steps a day

Taking an additional 2,000 steps throughout the day helps one maintain his or her weight, according to research by Dr. James O. Hill at the University of Colorado. Therefore, to lose weight, add in more steps.

⇀If you take 7,500 steps a day

7,500 steps a day was the cutting point for getting positive results for one workplace program. After 16 weeks, most employees who took at least 7,500 steps a day experienced improvement in quality of life, lost weight, felt more satisfied about their physical appearance, experienced positive feelings of self-esteem and increased confidence, and felt that their productivity had improved.

ACTIVE VIDEO-GAME PLAYING

Research shows that the energy expenditure for children during active screen time, playing particularly active video games, is on a par with moderate-intensity exercise. Energy expenditure increased two- to three-fold compared to television-watching. Heart rate also increased for those playing Wii boxing or DDR (Dance Dance Revolution) level 2, on a par with walking at a moderate rate. Wii bowling and beginner-level DDR created a twofold increase in energy expenditure compared to television-watching.

Improved balance was found among adults ages 61 to 89 who participated in active video games emphasizing balance, such as skiing. Those who played Wii bowling for 30 minutes burned an average of 103 calories, and 70 calories playing Wii baseball.

RESEARCH ON INCREASED STANDING TIMES

Researchers at the Take-A-Stand Project found that computer-users increased their standing time by 244%, or 66 minutes a day, when using the device that lifts the computer from a sitting position to a standing position. Employees reported improved moods and a 54% reduction in neck and back pain. Within two weeks of removing the devices, such gains were negated. It is reported that it is compulsory for employers to offer employees sit-stand desks in Denmark.

⇥If you take 8,000–10,000 steps a day
Taking 8,000-10,000 steps per day promotes weight loss.

⇥If you take 10,000 steps a day
Research shows that taking 10,000 steps a day over eight months can:
• Decrease waistline circumference by two inches.
• Result in weight loss of 10 pounds.
• Reduce high blood pressure by 34%.
• Decrease by 69% the odds for men of having cardiovascular disease.

Those who take 10,000 steps a day increase their insulin sensitivity by threefold when measured at five years, compared to those who take 3,000 steps a day. 35% report increase in confidence, which researchers infer reduces the likelihood of depression and anxiety. Research shows the impact on biomarkers as well.

Multi-tasking
Increase the value of the time you spend standing or walking by doing something as you move. Keep in mind that every action counts for your body's calorie expenditure, metabolism, and skeletal system.

IMPROVISING A STANDING STATION

A standing station can be anything that places your device at a convenient height for use while standing. You could try to improvise, using a fern stand for holding an iPad while watching TV, for example. For typing, a height that places your hands comfortably on a keyboard with elbows bent at a 90° is best. Use this as an opportunity to stand and/or walk in place on a reflexology mat.

Activities that provide a focus for doing something as one seeks to increase standing and walking time have benefits. Included are: expending more calories; setting the metabolism to a more natural setting; resisting insulin and leptin resistance, as well as making demands on the bones and muscles of the musculoskeletal system.

You can find the natural balance of activity in your day. Consider what research has found out about the following activities and what they can provide for you. Look for an activity that you like.

Using standing stations and desks

Sit-stand work stations

Office workers stand more during the day when they have access to a sit-stand device. The device holds the computer monitor and can be raised to a standing position.

The standing station

An opportunity to stand or move in place is created with a standing station. For use at home, the elevated surface can provide a convenient usable surface to hold a laptop, iPad, tablet, video game device, smartphone, or book.

The standing desk

More workers are standing at work using desks that adjust height to place computers and papers within convenient reach. Studies show increased calorie burning with the use

RESEARCH ON STANDING DESKS IN THE CLASSROOM

Offered use of a standing desk in one study, first-graders were enthusiastic about using them. Three-quarters of the students stood for 100% of the time they were at their desk, even though they were able to sit or stand as they pleased. In the study, conducted by Dr. Mark Benden of Texas A&M, first-graders in two classrooms who used standing desks expended 10 calories an hour or 17% more than those in two other classes who used traditional sitting desks during the school year. Overweight children expended an extra 23 calories an hour, or 32% more.

In further research Dr. Benden, an ergonomic engineer, found that children who were offered the standing desk with a stool did 12% better at "on-task engagement". As noted in a post by Christopher Bergland, "Benden said he wasn't surprised that the results of his recent study went beyond the calorie-burning benefits of standing. A wide range of studies have shown that even low levels of physical activity have a beneficial impact on cognitive ability."

"Standing workstations reduce disruptive behavior problems and increase students' attention or academic behavioral engagement by providing students with a different method for completing academic tasks (like standing) that breaks up the monotony of seated work," Benden said in a press release. "A standing desk can improve cognitive engagement and creative thinking. In other uses of the standing desk in the classroom, teachers report greater attentiveness, fewer behavioral problems, better posture and more enthusiasm. Kids who are habitually fidgety or who suffer from attention disorders appear to show the most improvement," teachers say.

of a standing desk. However, these desks are not without controversy. One researcher calls "standing at work 'one of the stupidest things one would ever want to do. This is the high heels of the furniture industry'." A group of researchers note the problems: long-term back injuries, increase in incidence of varicose veins, as well as increased heart beat.

Estimates vary, but use of a standing desk burns 20–35 calories more per hour than sitting in a desk chair. For those who sit five hours a day at work this adds up – to 100–165 calories per day. Not much, you might think, but consider this: researchers studied how much more sedentary jobs have become since 1970. They found the resulting lessened expenditure of calories to be 100 calories a day – enough to account for a significant portion of the increase in weight gain experienced by women and men in the US over the intervening years.

The treadmill desk

The treadmill desk is another way to create an active workplace, allowing you to work and be active at the same time. Using a treadmill desk or having one available for occasional use is reported to help employees be more alert and energetic. For one group of Air Force employees whose jobs are tied to equipment that cannot be left unattended, the use of the treadmill desk has resulted in them being more focused and productive, making fewer mistakes. In addition "complaints about the shift hours and the lack of sleep have virtually disappeared".

Acclimate yourself to a standing desk by using it for an hour a day to start off with, suggests Dr. Mark Bender. Then gradually build up more time.

Use of a treadmill desk consumes more calories. Dr. James Levine invented a treadmill desk and then tested it. He found that using a personal computer while walking at one mile an hour on a treadmill consumed 191 calories compared to the 72 calories of sitting in an office chair.

8 Enhanced walking techniques

If you're moving around more, why not enhance your efforts, getting more out of them? Where you walk and what's under your feet as you walk make a difference. Enhanced walking techniques provide heightened stimulation to the foot's sole or from the environment to boost the reflex value of your efforts.

Walking is more beneficial when it's in a green, leafy setting or barefoot on a surface of rock, bamboo, or pebbles. Biomarkers and other measures of health are positively impacted when walking in enhanced circumstances, when compared to those that aren't. What's going on?

The evolutionary design of the body includes a foot designed to be exposed to natural surfaces instead of encased in the sameness of a hard-soled, mass-manufactured shoe, worn on the uniform surfaces of sidewalks, streets, and indoor flooring. Stress is created on the finely tuned locomotive mechanism of the body, beginning with the foot. The reflex stimulation for which the foot is designed, to receive pressure sensation to its surface, with the foot as a whole designed to move and stretch in response to natural, uneven terrain, is limited.

Enhanced walking techniques provide an opportunity to mimic reflex actions lost to the modern-day person. Adding sensory experiences contributes "nutrition" to a reflex "diet".

Walking the reflex path

With reflexology path use, ancient tradition meets modern-day goals of health, fitness, and longevity. The paths that exist around the world consist of cobble or pebbles embedded or loosely placed in a sidewalk-like surface. You can try these out for yourself or improvise by walking on your own versions.

Walking on a cobblestone mat or real cobbles, if you have access to them, gives focus to your efforts to be up and about more. Knowing that you are receiving benefits beyond those you get from walking on a flat surface will provide you with the motivation to get moving around more.

Enhanced walking experiences are common in the Far East and seeing people walking barefoot on reflexology paths in city parks is a common sight across Asia. Visit a pharmacy in China and you'll be able to buy a mat with embedded plastic cobblestones to walk on at home when the weather is inclement.

Walking on a cobblestone mat or real cobbles gives focus to your efforts to be up and about more.

Most tap shek (stepping stone) paths in China are cobblestoned walkways and construction of these is part of the Chinese government's ten-year fitness plan. Along with funds to build athletic fields, money is put aside to build reflexology paths in parks to provide senior citizens and others with a moderate fitness activity, which is within their capabilities. Considering it a "fashionable fitness activity", Chinese seniors line up in city parks twice a day for their 15-minute walks and when it rains, they have the option of staying at home and walking on their own reflexology mats. Found throughout Asia are mats and devices with textured surfaces on which to walk and a whole industry has built up around the manufacture and sale of them.

Japanese "reflex therapy promenades" are designed with each sidewalk-like segment designed to have a carefully crafted surface that works on a specific part of the foot. The paths are found in city parks, nature parks, fitness facilities, natural hot-spring spas, business parks, and even in a car-park garage and on the roof of a sewage-treatment plant. In some instances the paths are built into theme parks with hot springs and/or facilities for traditional bathing.

In Germany and Austria, "Barfusspads" (barefoot paths) are designed so that you can go on a hike of several kilometers through a forest with your bare feet making contact with specifically selected and positioned natural surfaces. The paths include natural elements such as bark, logs, stones, moss, and mud. Water features with textured walking surfaces offer an aquatic experience by way of variation.

Some 20 city parks in Seoul include "barefoot shiatsu courses", which offer opportunities for an "eco-experience". Botanical gardens are designed to mimic a forest or nature as experienced while walking on "manicured" barefoot shiatsu courses. The general purposes of barefoot walking is to allow you to feel a sense of unity with nature to relieve accumulated stress and also to acquire the positive thinking necessary to bring about psychological and spiritual healing. This, in turn, will lead to overall healing, health, and relief from general tiredness.

How walking reflexology works
According to Chinese reports, walking on a cobblestoned surface exposes more of the foot to a surface than walking on a flat surface. When the soles of the feet are stimulated in this way, the postural muscles are affected and results include: controlled muscle contraction and relaxation, squeezed peripheral vascular muscles, expanded blood vessels, reduced high blood pressure, promotion of the body's insulin secretion, improved blood circulation, lower cholesterol, promotion of the body metabolism, and enhanced immune function. These results occur because of improved circulation with stimulation of the peripheral nerves and acupuncture points, speeded-up blood flow, greatly increased oxygen consumption, producing a specialized vessel wall, cleaning particles of fat and cholesterol.

RESEARCH ON REFLEXOLOGY PATHS AND MATS

American researchers attending a conference in Shanghai became intrigued with reflexology paths when they saw people walking on one in a city park there. Researchers John Fischer, Fuzhong Li, and Peter Harmer of the Oregon Research Institute came home and conducted a study to see if the traditional use of the paths for health could be verified by research.

Study results showed that compared to those who walked on a flat surface, the mat-walkers experienced significantly reduced pain and diastolic blood pressure; greatly improved perceptions of control over falls; significantly reduced daytime sleepiness; increased psychosocial wellbeing, and considerable improvements in ability to perform the usual activities of daily living.

"Cobblestone mat walking (three times a week for 45 minutes over eight weeks) improved physical function and reduced blood pressure to a greater extent than conventional walking in older adults. Additional benefits of this walking program included improved health-related quality of life. This new physical activity may provide a therapeutic and health-enhancing exercise alternative for older adults."

The results prompted the researchers to call mat-walking "enhanced walking".

Reducing blood pressure

Compared to a consistent program of conventional walking on a flat surface, reflex mat-walking accelerated the lowering of long-term, average diastolic blood pressure.

Two ORI (Oregon Research Institute) studies demonstrated that study participants who walked on a reflex mat for 45 minutes three times per week for four months showed diastolic blood pressure to be lowered by 4.75 points, compared to those who walked the same time and distance on a flat surface.

Studies have shown that walking 10,000 steps a day (two and a half hours of walking at a normal pace throughout the day) for three months lowered participants' diastolic blood pressure by eight points. When the time spent walking is compared, long-term average blood pressure is, thus, lowered seven times faster using mat-walking.

The use of reflexology paths benefits an individual and widespread use would provide societal impact, including affecting hypertension, which is a major risk factor for heart disease and stroke, according to a Chinese website.

Avoiding falls

ORI research showed, in comparison to those who practiced "conventional walking" during the study, mat-walking participants reported "significant improvement in their ability to control falling". Falls are "the leading cause of long term disability, premature institutionalization and injury-related deaths in the older population".

Multiple studies indicate falls and other gait problems may be an early indicator of Alzheimer's. Improvement through mat-walking may help reduce risk of falls and influence the risk of Alzheimer's.

Potential exists for using such paths to encourage increased physical activity over a broad population and, thus, impact and

PERFECT FOR BUSINESS PEOPLE

For employer Shiseido in Japan use of the company's reflexology path by employees resulted in improvements in productivity, sick leave, and, over time, health-care costs. For employees the reflexology path is a 15-minute, 75-meter barefooted walk on a sidewalk-like surface surrounded by green grass, trees, and a picnic table. Materials underfoot vary from segment to segment and include gravel, embedded rock, and halved bamboo, targeting specific parts of the foot associated with certain reflex areas, are placed in sidewalk-like sections, some of which are repeated over the course of the path.

lessen risks for dementia and Alzheimer's. Research shows physical inactivity is calculated to represent 21% of lifestyle contributions to the risk for Alzheimer's. The ORI study showed cobblestone mat-walking to be an answer to the quest for "simple, convenient, and readily accessible exercise programs that will reduce health problems and improve quality of life of the aging population". Also, study participants reported they enjoyed the activity, would recommend it to friends and would continue if possible. Cobblestone path-walking throughout Asia shows possibility for "societal level interventions" to increase physical activity.

Losing weight: a "functional diet"
The small movement of stepping-stone walking is seen as a "functional diet" with weight loss taking place as functions of the body improve over time as you walk on a cobblestoned surface. It is seen to produce a "diet effect" because stimulation of the peripheral nerves of the feet conditions the nerve and endocrine function as well as regulation of the appetite, reducing it and increasing satiety.

Cited in Chinese articles are researchers who report results including: conditioning the regulation of appetite and satiety;

RESEARCH ON BEAD MAT-WALKING

The speed of blood circulation was doubled following a five-minute walk on a beaded mat. Research by Tauro Nakamura found that other changes included improved surface temperature of the foot and improved indicators of sympathetic nervous system activity.

Ultrasonic measurements were used to test the speed of blood circulation. The average before measurement was 12.5 centimeters per second with an after measurement of 29.0 cm per second. Measurements using thermography found that bead mat-walking improved the surface temperature of the foot and and more evenly distributed it over the foot. The response of the autonomic nervous system to mat-walking was measured by change in electrical resistance using Galvanic skin response.

MAKE YOUR OWN REFLEXOLOGY MAT

A contest run by a Chinese magazine produced a winning idea for creating a reflexology mat. Take a large bag, such as one onions come in, and place rocks in it in a shallow layer. Flatter rocks are less challenging than three-dimensional ones. Close the bag and place it on a carpet, rug, or yoga mat, and walk across it.

improving blood circulation; and aiding in the metabolism of fats. It is said stepping-stone walking stimulates acupuncture points simultaneously, but also regulates nerve and endocrine function, inhibition of the brain regulates appetite of the nerve, reduces appetite, increases satiety, and thus plays a diet effect. It is suggested that 30 minutes of stepping-stone fitness per day reduces the appetite by half. Stepping-stone walking of 30 minutes a day over the period of a year is noted as having "been tested by experts" and found to have the potential for a weight loss of 20 pounds.

DON'T USE A COBBLESTONE PATH IF …

If you suffer from osteoporosis, arthritis, foot injury, foot infection, plantar fascitis, diabetes, neuropathy, bone and knee degenerations you should consult a physician. The elderly and those with musculoskeletal problems should consider how long and how often to walk on a cobblestone path. Walking more frequently for a shorter time may help avoid discomfort. Chinese seniors walk 15 minutes twice a day because of such concerns.

Beaded mat-walking

Warmer feet, better circulation, and impact on the autonomic nervous system were found with participants in a Japanese study of walking on a beaded mat.

Bamboo stepping: aotake

Aotake (bamboo-stepping) is a Japanese tradition that dates back to the times of the samurai. The warriors are reported to have chopped off a piece of bamboo and then walked on it to improve their stamina – the tradition continues in Japan today. In some situations, the rounded sides of halved bamboo, spaced the distance of a footstep, form the walking surface. In other situations, participants walk in place on halved bamboo or a variety of rounded plastic, knobby-surfaced devices. To try this out for yourself, place a broom on the floor and try stepping on the handle.

Reduce stress

Research shows that the use of bamboo-stepping helps reduce stress and stress-related problems. Pediatric-care nurses in Japan sought to help reduce stress among mothers staying with their hospitalized children and bamboo-stepping was introduced. It was successful because it could be used anywhere.

Reduced nausea and vomiting

Studying the effect of bamboo-stepping on cancer patients who were receiving chemotherapy, Chinese researchers found that 20 to 30 minutes, three times daily, of bamboo-stepping significantly reduced nausea and vomiting following chemotherapy for 62.5% of study participants and was effective for 28%.

Barefoot education is thought to encourage development of the brain by stimulating the senses.

Improved learning and development

"Barefoot education", or elementary schools with shoeless students, is not an uncommon phenomenon in Japan since barefoot education is thought to encourage development of the brain by stimulating the senses. A bamboo-walking surface spaced the distance of a footstep is featured in children's playgrounds to use during play and physical education. Halved bamboo is fixed into the floor, spaced the distance of a footstep, on half the walking surfaces of school hallways.

Improved mood

A step exercise program for senior citizens using a plastic, textured bar simulating bamboo has proven to be popular in Japan. Researchers found that the 40-minute program provided at health clubs brought about significant changes in negative mood states such as tension, anger, fatigue, depression, and confusion.

THE AOTAKE STEP EXERCISE PROGRAM

The Aotake program has become very popular as an age-appropriate activity for senior citizens. It involves low-impact aerobics, no equipment other than an inexpensive Aotake step, easy-to-learn dance steps, enjoyable music, and reflex stimulation. Participants move in time to the music, stepping onto a plastic strip about 2½ inches high, 16 inches long, and 3 inches wide. The strip is textured with raised bumps, which provide reflex stimulation thought by many to promote relaxation and balance throughout the body.

WEARING MASSAGE SANDALS

Several brands of massage sandals are available, so try before you buy – to see if you like them. Start by wearing them for a short time, allowing yourself to become acclimated. Alternatively, wear them with socks. The heavier the socks, the more protective they will be of your foot and the less challenge the sandals will be.

Massage sandals

Massage sandals provide an enhanced standing and walking experience through having a textured sole bed. They are available in different levels of challenge, with sole beds ranging from small bumps, to pronged nodules, to stone sandals.

Research demonstrates the potential for enhancement of simply standing or walking around wearing these sandals. In a collaborative study between the Kenkoh sandal company and the University of Kyoto Graduate School of Medicine, results were compared for study participants who walked around for four hours wearing a pronged Kenkoh sandal to those who wore a smooth sole bed version. Those who wore the pronged version experienced a decrease in diastolic blood pressure, systolic blood pressure, and pulse rate. Pronged-sandal wearers also reported decrease in tiredness; less listlessness; decrease in tired feet; lessened pain in the soles of the feet; foot warmth; improved mood, good mood; body warmth and comfort; and sensations of body lightness. It is thought that the sandals "promote" blood flow back to the heart as well as emulate results provided by shiatsu and reflexology practices.

Forest "bathing" and "medicine"

A walk in the forest is a pleasant experience anyway, but extensive research shows that forest "bathing" or "medicine" has health benefits. Walking in a forest environment prompts reflexive responses with benefits not only from walking but also from experiencing the sights, sounds, smells, and tactile sensations of the forest. These sensory experiences impact physiological and psychological responses as they tap into our innate, inherent reflex responses to a natural setting.

For years Japanese researchers have studied the health-enhancing impact of walking in the forest. Shinrin-yoku, or "taking in the forest atmosphere or forest bathing", was coined by the Japanese Ministry of Agriculture, Forestry, and Fisheries in 1982. It has now become a recognized relaxation and/or stress-management activity in Japan. Researchers found that health benefits include lowered blood pressure, lowered blood-glucose levels, increased activities of the immune system, and improvements in biomarkers related to fat and sugar metabolism as well as stress reduction.

RESEARCH ON FOREST-BATHING

Forest-bathing is a recognized relaxation and stress-management activity in Japan. According to Japanese researchers, habitual forest-bathing may lower the risk of stress-related disorders.

In one study, researchers compared measures of physiological and psychological stress for young men who spent three days and two nights in a forest setting and the same amount of time in an urban setting. Stress-related markers were taken, including heart-rate variability, blood pressure, pulse rate, ECG, salivary cortisol, and salivary amylase.

The results of heart-rate variability analysis showed that the forest environment created a significant shift to a "... greater parasympathetic activity and lower sympathetic nerve activity than do city environments". Changes in others measured indicated increased relaxation. Psychological tests showed a significant increase in positive feelings and a decrease in negative feelings.

They note the broad implications include the possible use of forest-bathing to reduce health-care costs, to reduce stress, and lower blood pressure, decreasing the risk of "psychosocial stress-related diseases". Research showed that a forest walk increased activities of the immune system for healthy volunteers, acting as a "cancer preventive", according to researchers, with effects lasting for three weeks.

Why would this happen? "Forest environments affect humans via the five senses, providing stimulation of various senses, such as vision (scenery), olfaction (smell of wood), audition (sound of running streams or the rustle of leaves), tactile sensation (feel of

NO FOREST NEARBY?

While Japanese researchers note the benefits of exposure to forest-bathing, walking through a densely planted city park is seen to provide benefit. Other researchers have detailed the benefits of being exposed to nature when working in a garden. Even five minutes of exercise in a green space provides positive mental effects. Water in the green space provides an even bigger boost.

Just looking at a green scene from a window lowers the blood pressure and pulse rate as well as improve mood and level of cortisol. A hospital window with a view of trees speeds recovery for heart patients. Looking at a picture of green trees including water is calming and living near a green space creates health benefits. Other researchers have found benefits in the virtual reality of viewing a computer-generated natural environment for 10 minutes.

Then there are indoor benefits of reflex responses to nature and natural materials to be found. Being in a room with wood on 30% of the surfaces creates a significantly decreased pulse rate and diastolic blood pressure.

the surfaces of trees and leaves). Sensory information inputs via the five senses are processed in the corresponding sensory areas of the brain and are further transmitted through interaction among the various sensory inputs."

Forest medicine or forest-bathing, immersing yourself in the sensory-rich environment of a forest when walking, is a popular activity throughout Asia. In Seoul, Korea, the two ideas are merged with "barefoot shiatsu courses" available in city parks that are landscaped to mimic a forest. Visits for a walk in forested national parks in mountainous areas include opportunities for forest-bathing and barefoot walking ("barefoot shiatsu"), wildflower-viewing, birding, and photography. Barefoot walking in scenic surroundings as a part of "forest-bathing" is seen to help you enjoy nature, ease fatigue, relax stress, and ease feet accustomed to walking on hard surfaces.

Effects of forest-bathing

Blood pressure

A forest experience of walking for 15 minutes and observing nature for 15 minutes created a significantly lower blood pressure and heart rate for study participants as compared to a city walking experience.

Metabolic syndrome/risk for heart attack

Compared to a two-hour walk in the city, a two-hour walk in a forest showed significant effect on several indicators associated with reduced risk of heart attack as well as elements of metabolic syndrome according to Japanese researchers.

Cancer preventive

A three-day, two-night visit to a forest area created results described as a "cancer preventive" by Japanese researchers. The effects lasted 30 days and were not seen during a three-day/two-night city visit.

Similar results were also seen from a study of an eight-hour visit to a forest by participants.

Cardiac preventive

Elderly hypertensive patients who spent seven days and seven nights in a forest environment experienced therapeutic benefits while such benefits were not experienced during a city visit. Tested were blood pressure and C-reactive protein. The Chinese researchers note that forest bathing has therapeutic effects as a "natural therapy for human hypertension".

Glucose tolerance/insulin sensitivity/diabetes

Compared to their pre-walk levels, blood-glucose levels measured significantly lower for type-two diabetics after a three- or six-kilometer walk in the forest. Writing about significantly lowered blood-glucose levels, Japanese researchers noted, "The authors concluded that Shinrin-yoku (forest bathing) was useful in the treatment of diabetes mellitus."

Depression

Compared to going about their usual daily activities, spending the day in a forest showed a significant change of mood, with a decrease in depression and hostility, while "liveliness" increased significantly for study participants.

9 Systems to feed your reflexes

It's possible you're already supercharging your standing, walking, and moving reflexes if you practice reflexology, yoga, or tai chi. These systems provide an opportunity to unconsciously "feed" your body the right "nutrition", the standing, walking, and moving "nutrients" it needs to maintain your body.

People who practice reflexology, yoga, and tai chi report a sense of relaxation and calm transcending the physical realm, resulting in pain reduction, improved gait, and a lessened fear of falls, for example. But breaking the routine of sitting can be enhanced even further using these systems. If you are using the discipline of standing up every 20 minutes, for example, it can easily become regimented and tedious, but systems such as reflexology, yoga, and tai chi add interest and many important benefits. If you find a practice that suits you, you may well find that you become a lifelong follower of it.

How reflex systems work
Reflex systems provide exercise of a fuller range of proprioceptive mechanisms that interact with the inner "you". Proprioceptors are sensors that help our bodies know where they are in three-dimensional space and what they are doing in real time. Proprioceptive information, referred to as the "sixth sense", includes sensing deep pressure to the bottoms of the feet, the stretch of muscles, and angulation of joints.

REFLEXOLOGY, YOGA, AND TAI CHI

What are the essential points to note about the three disciplines?

→ Reflexology is the systematic application of pressure to reflex areas on the hands and feet by yourself or another, for the purpose of affecting other parts of the body
→ Yoga is a system of postures that strengthens the body, engaging mind, body, and spirit
→ Tai chi is a soft martial art, engaging the body in flowing movement and shifting energy

As proprioceptive activities take place, they stimulate automatic and unconscious responses of our body's metabolism, the fats, sugars, and other ingredients that fuel our movements. The activities of the autonomic nervous system, brain, and the musculoskeletal system are affected as well.

Cave-dwelling people didn't go to gyms, they didn't need them; their entire world was a gym and they experienced a fuller range of the body's proprioceptive potential. Reflexology, yoga, and tai chi enthusiasts are today responding to something that their bodies need and a lack we all experience in the modern age: a sharpening of reflexes, and more, which is not provided in daily life. Each practice creates change in the operation of the inner "you" and impacts lifestyle conditions. The result is improvements in instinctual abilities to move and balance as well as better core muscle performance.

Sedentary living translates into a body that has lessened reflexive stability and instinctual abilities to perform basic movements. Andrew Heffernan, writing in *Men's Health*, notes that even 120 years ago people engaged in a greater variety of daily physical activities than we do today. Even those who routinely exercise tend to perform the same kinds of physical activities over and over again, so they lack all-round stimulation.

The benefits of the systems

Reflexology, yoga, and tai chi provide a systematic approach to pressure, stretch, and movement activities that stimulate the core muscles of the body and/or the sensors in the feet. Among the benefits is substituting active time for sitting time. The results are similar to those found in a light-intensity physical activity with impact on metabolism but with expanded benefits. Aside from reducing blood pressure, for example, tai chi improves gait for senior citizens. Reflexology and yoga lessen musculoskeletal pain. Just as with any reflex "diet" technique, the key to obtaining results using the reflex systems is the appropriate "dose": how much, how often, and how intense?

Reflexology

Reflexology's techniques are used to systematically apply pressure to the feet. Pressure is a key signal that we're not sitting, which is central to postural muscle activation and activity of the inner "you". Pressure perceived by the feet as we stand and walk makes a difference to how our bodies operate. Targeted are reflex areas that mirror parts of the body.

WHAT IS REFLEXOLOGY?

Reflexology is the systematic application of pressure to the feet, providing information to the sensors that make walking possible. Linking the foot's pressure information and the inner "you" is the need to coordinate activities of the body. In case of danger, for example, the feet participate in an overall body reaction known as "fight or flight". As the body prepares its internal structure to provide for either eventuality, muscles ready for action are a part of this overall body response. In case of danger, the hands reach for a weapon and the feet prepare to fight or flee.

This same mechanism is at work 24/7. Pressure perceived by the feet helps set the activity of the inner "you".

THE BENEFITS OF DOING REFLEXOLOGY

Reflexology has been shown to benefit the body in the following different ways:

→ Decrease in blood pressure
→ Marked difference in cholesterol
→ Lessened fear of falling for those who use reflexology mats
→ Reduced fasting glucose levels for diabetics
→ Pain reduction
→ Decease in triglycerides in those who are hypertensive

Reflexology practices are found in ancient civilizations and modern Asian practices mirror this heritage. Current Western practices emerged from European and Russian research into the nervous system and the reflex – think Pavlov and his dogs.

Reflexology application can be used for many kinds of wellbeing, but in particular stress reduction. Techniques provide a variety of sensory experiences and demands that interrupt the patterns of stress created by walking. The foot is used as a keyboard to ask the body to interrupt its stress programming and pay attention to the demands of pressure technique application. Through practice of the foot's full capabilities, stress can be interrupted. With consistent application, the body can be conditioned to adapt to stress in the most positive ways and ongoing application creates an educational experience.

Reflexology interrupts the cycle of stress by creating a set of demands on the body separate from everyday experiences. Its goal is to apply pressure techniques to interrupt stress and provoke response within the dynamics of the stress mechanism. In addition, over time, the stress mechanism is conditioned to behave in a manner that creates less wear and tear on the body. The pressure techniques of reflexology are applied by a practitioner or you can apply them yourself.

Yoga

The 5,000-year-old practice of yoga includes exercise, breathing, and meditation. Here we consider it as a practice of reflexes that are important to walking and standing. Some cite yoga as helping body alignment that has been put under stress by sitting.

Holding even a minute-long yoga posture lowers the stress hormone cortisol and raises prolactin and oxytocin, the feel-good hormones, and studies show that three-weekly 20-minute sessions can enhance blood flow in your arteries. It can relax chronic muscle tension and, through diaphragmatic breathing, improve oxygen absorption. Yoga works to balance the two parts of the nervous system: the stress-response sympathetic unit and the parasympathetic part, which maintains your wellbeing.

Tai Chi

Tai chi is an ancient practice of controlled movements and meditation. Research shows that the discipline impacts lifestyle conditions and gait. The practice of tai chi appears to work in part within some of the same mechanisms that provide benefits when one exercises. As noted by one study comparing participants who walked and those who practiced tai chi, "In general the stress-reduction effect of Tai Chi characterized moderate physical exercise. Heart rate, blood pressure, and urinary catecholamine changes for Tai Chi were found to be similar to those for walking at a speed of 6km/hr."

Mindfulness

At the center of mindfulness is awareness. Here we are concerned about being aware of the effect of what you do on your body. Remember, for the hotel maids, becoming aware of what they did and how their bodies' activities impacted changed their perceptions and functioning.

Everything you take for granted – the sitting, standing, and walking that impact the inner "you" – you can add a mindful element to it for your benefit. For example, mindfulness and

WHAT IS YOGA?

Yoga is an ancient discipline focusing on "asanas", or postures, which can either flow or be static, depending on the style. Breathing techniques can also be employed and the discipline has a meditative and spiritual focus. The body works with itself towards strengthening, by holding positions for varying amounts of time. Through this, the mind is also strengthened and ultimately the practitioner can access spiritual depths. Regular practice brings about fitness, suppleness, health, healing, and mental peace.

THE BENEFITS OF DOING YOGA

Yoga has been shown to benefit the body in the following ways:

→ Lowered blood pressure
→ Lowered cholesterol
→ Reduction in triglycerides
→ Reduced fasting glucose levels for diabetics
→ Pain reduction
→ Reduced waist circumference and weight loss

WHAT IS TAI CHI?

Tai chi is a "soft martial art", originating in China, practiced largely for the benefits it can give personal health – especially strength and balance, connecting mind, body, and spirit. It is a slow-moving "form", which creates a seamless flow of movement that the practitioner memorizes. Energy, or chi, is moved around and between the limbs via energy meridians in the body.

THE BENEFITS OF DOING TAI CHI

Tai chi has been shown to benefit the body in the following ways:

- Decreased blood pressure
- Reduction in bad cholesterol and increase in good cholesterol
- Reduced fasting glucose levels for diabetics
- Lessened fear of falling and improvements in balance in senior practitioners
- Pain reduction for arthritis
- Exercise value
- Reduced symptoms for ADHD adolescents
- Weight control

eating leads one to pay attention to the food, its texture, taste, how you eat it, and the whole culinary experience.

Sitting is an activity we carry out with little thought or focus. To reverse this trend one can practice mindfulness techniques such as when you sit down and how long you sit for. Also, what happens as you sit? Do you feel discomfort in your muscles and joints? At some point do you start fidgeting, moving uncomfortably about?

Consider changing your awareness of sitting as a benign activity and replacing it with a real image of what your body is going through. You're moving sitting from being a subconscious activity to a conscious one. Instead of turning off your senses, you're turning them on. You feel the chair against your body and experience its softness or hardness. Be aware of your posture and the position of your body. As you sit, over time, what is the effect on your muscles, your joints, and your mood? Are you happy with what's going on? Where is your tipping point concerning when you feel the need to get up and move?

Try out all the chairs you sit on throughout the day. How do they compare? What is your favorite chair? Do you sit upright or do you slouch? Recline in a recliner? Are you conscious of your body as you sit? Mindful sitting is tuning in to the wholeness of the experience. Be aware, also, of the impact on your muscles, nerves, and skin.

Now consider how aware you are of your body as you stand or walk. Try walking around the house in your bare feet. Consider what's underfoot and how it feels. Note the difference between a soft rug and a hard surface. Do you move your arms as you walk? Try drawing your body up straight, as tall as you can. Suck your stomach in. Now walk. Put on your everyday work shoes and walk around. How do your feet feel now?

10 Reflex solutions and summary

You are what you do and what you spend your time doing. But how much of which activities creates what effects? Reflex solutions provide you with the answers.

Here are the reflex techniques and the amounts of time linked to decrease the risk of abnormal biomarkers, indicators, or lifestyle concerns. Noted, in some cases, as well are the reflex activities that increase risk. Following the "recipe for success" minimum dose will provide you with your basic "diet". Reflex solutions provide information so that you can be mindful of how what you do impacts the inner cave-dweller "you".

Note that the following includes categories of television-watching time and screen time. The results indicated are for uninterrupted seated time. Results in the sitting-time category are for uninterrupted sitting time.

Metabolic biomarkers and other indicators

Metabolic biomarkers and other indicators are measurements of how the inner cave-dweller "you" is working. They are also the building blocks of chronic degenerative lifestyle conditions. How sitting creates an effect on them is discussed in Chapter 3 and how to influence them is discussed here.

Blood pressure

Elevated blood pressure is an indicator for: cardiovascular disease, stroke, heart attack, cognitive decline, dementia, Alzheimer's disease, obesity, and metabolic syndrome.

Reflex activities that increase risk for elevated blood pressure

➥ Television-watching time
  - Sitting more than four hours per day during time off while watching television increased by 55% the odds of higher blood pressure for men compared to sitting watching television for less than one hour per day.

➥ Sitting
  - For half of the women in one study sitting significantly increased blood pressure. Lack of muscle tone in the legs, causing their hearts to work harder to return blood from the extremities, was thought to be the reason.

Reflex techniques that decrease risk for elevated blood pressure

➥ Take 10,000 steps
  - Walking 10,000 steps (approximately five miles) over the course of a day for over four months reduced high blood pressure by 34%.
  - Walking 10,000 steps a day for 12 weeks lowered diastolic blood pressure by 8 points.

➥ Take breaks in sitting
  - Taking two-minute breaks in sitting every 20 minutes over seven hours lowered blood pressure by three points.
  - Standing up for 90 seconds lowered blood pressure.

➥ Consider trying the electric foot-vibrating platform solution.
  - Blood pressure remained normal for those using an electric foot-vibrating platform, mitigating the effects on blood pressure of prolonged sitting.

➥ Consider the cobblestone mat-walking solution
  - Walking on a cobblestone mat three times a week for 45 minutes over four months lowered diastolic blood pressure by 4.75 points.

➥ Consider the rocking-chair solution
  • Thirty minutes of steady rocking in a rocking chair led to an increase of systolic blood pressure of 12–20 points and a 2.5–3.6 points average increase in diastolic blood pressure, normalizing the extreme drop in blood pressure experienced by some during sitting.
➥ Consider the reflexology solution
  • Blood pressure lowered by 25 points using reflexology over 30–40 days, commensurate with that of the study participants on medication.
➥ Consider the tai chi solution
  • One hour of tai chi three times per week for 12 weeks was associated with significant improvements in systolic and diastolic blood pressure.
➥ Consider the yoga solution
  • Yoga practiced for four weeks to 12 months lowered diastolic blood pressure 4.9% to 24.2% and systolic blood pressure 2.6% to 21.3%.
➥ Consider the massage sandal-wearing solution
  • Wearing Kenkoh massage sandals for four hours while moving about reduced systolic blood pressure (12%), diastolic blood pressure (6%) as well as lowering pulse rate (18%)
➥ Consider the forest-bathing solution
  • Walking and sitting in a forest for 15 minutes each created significantly lower blood pressure and heart rate compared to walking and sitting in an urban area.

Cholesterol

Elevated cholesterol levels are an indicator for: cardiovascular disease, stroke, heart attack, cognitive decline, Alzheimer's disease, obesity, and metabolic syndrome.

Reflex activities that increase risk for abnormal cholesterol (HDL-C) levels

➥ Screen-watching time
  • The number of hours of television-viewing were significantly associated with increased low-density lipoprotein (bad)

cholesterol as well as lessened HDL (good) cholesterol.
  • Men who sat and watched television or used the computer outside of work hours for more than four hours had double the odds of low "good" cholesterol (HDL-C) compared to those who did so for less than one hour.
  • More than two hours per day of television-viewing increased the risk of abnormal concentrations of cholesterol.
→ Sitting time
  • Those who sat the most had poorer indicators for cholesterol compared to those who sat the least.

Reflex techniques that decrease risk for abnormal cholesterol (HDL-C) levels

→ Take lifestyle steps
  • For every 1,000 steps taken during lifestyle activities of daily living reduced risk of low HDL by 12%. Taking steps every 30 minutes reduced risk of low HDL by 11%.
→ Take breaks in sitting
  • Even one minute of standing made a difference, resulting in lower levels of HDL ("good") cholesterol.
  • Those who took the most breaks in sitting had the best profiles for fats.
→ Consider the reflexology solution
  • Reflexology applied 30 to 40 minutes daily for 12 days in one study and for 20 sessions in another resulted in a marked statistical difference in cholesterol.
→ Consider the yoga solution
  • Yoga practice in amounts of six weeks to 12 months reduced total cholesterol by 5.8% to 25.2% and bad cholesterol by 12.8% to 26.0%.
→ Consider the tai chi solution
  • A six-month program of kung fu or tai chi was related to reduction in total cholesterol for overweight adolescents.

C-reactive protein

C-reactive protein is an indicator of low-grade inflammation associated with risk for cardiovascular disease, cancer, and other lifestyle conditions.

Reflex activities that increase risk for elevated C-reactive protein levels

➥ Screen-viewing time
- Approximately twice the level of C-reactive protein was found in those who sat for more than four hours per day during non-work screen time. The levels were three times higher in those who spent more than six hours in front of a screen.

➥ Sitting time
- More sitting time is significantly associated with increased C-reactive protein levels according to cancer researchers.
- The more the sitting time, the higher the level of C-reactive protein.

Reflex techniques that decrease risk for elevated C-reactive protein levels

➥ Take lifestyle steps
- Light-intensity physical activity is associated with reduced C-reactive protein levels.

➥ Take breaks in sitting
- A break of even one minute makes a difference in levels of C-reactive protein. One study showed that those who took the most breaks in sitting had reduced levels of C-reactive protein.

➥ Consider the forest-bathing solution
- Seven days and seven nights in a forest environment created therapeutic benefits, a reduction in C-reactive protein.

➥ Consider the tai chi solution
- A six-month program of kung fu or tai chi resulted in decreased C-reactive protein for overweight adolescents

Diabetes prevention/glucose/blood sugar/ glucose tolerance/insulin sensitivity/insulin resistance

Research demonstrates the effects of prolonged sitting on glucose, insulin, and risk for diabetes. Sugar metabolism (glucose, blood sugar, glucose tolerance, insulin sensitivity, insulin resistance) is an indicator for cardiovascular disease, stroke, heart attack, cognitive decline, dementia, Alzheimer's disease, cancer, diabetes, obesity, metabolic syndrome.

Physical inactivity is estimated to be the main cause for approximately 27% of diabetes. More than 25% of Americans over the age of 65 have type-two diabetes. An additional 50% are pre-diabetic.

Reflex activities that increase risk for elevated glucose levels
→ Sitting time
  • Those who sat two hours more a day (men) and 1½ hours (women) experienced an 18% worsened glucose level.
  • Each two-hour per day increment in sitting at work is associated with a 7% increase in diabetes.
→ Taking fewer steps
  • Blood-sugar levels spiked by 26% for those walking less than 3,000 steps a day compared to 10,000 steps a day.
→ Television-watching time
  • Each two hours of television-watching resulted in a 20% increase in risk for type-two diabetes.
  • Men who watched television between three and six hours a day had twice the risk of developing diabetes. Men who watched more than six hours a day were three times as likely to develop diabetes.
→ Screen-viewing time
  • A 32% higher odds of elevated glucose was seen in men who sat watching television and/or using the computer outside working hours for more than four hours per day.
  • Men aged 20 to 38 who engaged in the greatest number of hours of watching television and using a computer had a 2.5-fold increase in risk for insulin resistance.
  • More than two hours per day of television-viewing increased the risk of insulin resistance.

Reflex techniques that decrease risk for elevated glucose levels
→ Take breaks in sitting
  • Taking frequent small breaks for as little as one minute in

prolonged sitting makes a significant difference in sugar metabolism.

- A break in sitting of two minutes every 20 minutes normalizes the processing of sugars after eating. Important for heart health and avoiding risk for cardiovascular disease, metabolic syndrome, and diabetes.
- Each hour of light physical activity (cooking, washing dishes, ironing, and other routine domestic or occupational tasks) done while standing or walking decreased glucose levels by 16% over a week.
- A 24% reduction in glucose levels resulted when middle-aged women engaged in 15 or 40 minutes of light-intensity physical activity.

➥ Consider light-physical-intensity activity, moderate-to-vigorous physical intensity
- The less the light, moderate, and/or vigorous physical activity, the higher the insulin-resistance level.

➥ Consider the electric foot vibrator, foot-roller, and foot-bath solution
- Use of an electric foot-vibrating platform, an electric foot roller, or a foot bath significantly improves heart-rate variability, the interval between heart beats. Decreased heart-rate variability is associated with a sedentary lifestyle as well as increased risk of type-two diabetes and insulin resistance.

➥ Consider the forest-bathing solution
- A three- or six-kilometer walk in the forest resulted in significantly lower blood-glucose levels for type-two diabetes study participants.
- A two-hour walk in the morning and the afternoon significantly increased levels of the hormone adiponectin, which enhances insulin sensitivity and glucose tolerance.

➥ Consider the reflexology solution
- Reflexology applied daily for 30 days greatly reduced fasting glucose levels for diabetic patients.

➥ Consider the tai chi solution
- A six-month program of kung fu or tai chi resulted in reductions in insulin resistance for overweight adolescents.

- One hour of tai chi three times per week for 12 weeks was associated with significant improvements in insulin resistance.
- Supervised tai chi practice twice a week with self-practice three times a week at home over six months significantly lowered fasting blood-glucose levels for individuals with diabetes.

➡ Consider the yoga solution
- Multiple yoga studies demonstrate improvements in measurements of insulin resistance following 40 days to 12 months of practice.

Leptin/leptin resistance

Leptin is a protein released into the bloodstream by fat cells as they fill with triglyceride. Circulation in the blood through the body's appestat, the hypothalamus of the brain, is an indicator for how much fat is in storage and whether the body needs to take in more food. It is a biomarker for cardiovascular disease, obesity, Alzheimer's disease, and other disorders.

Reflex activities that increase risk for elevated leptin levels/leptin resistance

➡ Television-watching time
- Hours of television watching were significantly associated with decreased levels of leptin in research including 468 healthy male health professionals as participants, followed over six years.

➡ Sitting time
- Sitting time was associated with leptin levels in women.

Reflex activities that potentially decrease risk for elevated leptin levels/leptin resistance

➡ Lessen television-watching and sitting time

Lipoprotein lipase

Lipoprotein lipase (LPL) is an enzyme released by postural muscles as they move to draw fat from the bloodstream into the muscles. It is an indicator linked to a myriad lifestyle conditions:

atherosclerosis, obesity, Alzheimer's disease, metabolic syndrome, and a condition associated with diabetes and insulin resistance.

Reflex activities that increase risk for abnormal lipoprotein lipase levels
⇀ Sitting time
  · LPL levels drop by 50% after a day of sitting.

Reflex techniques that potentially decrease risk for abnormal lipoprotein lipase levels
⇀ Take breaks in sitting and lessen sitting time

Triglycerides
Triglyceride levels are indicators for cardiovascular disease, stroke, and heart attack; cognitive decline; obesity, and metabolic syndrome.

Reflex activities that increase risk for elevated triglyceride levels
⇀ Television-watching time
  · More than two hours per day of television-viewing increased risk of elevated triglyceride levels.

Reflex techniques that decrease risk for elevated triglyceride levels
⇀ Take breaks in sitting
  · Even a one-minute break in sitting made a difference in triglyceride levels.
⇀ Take steps
  · Every 1,000 steps reduced the risk of elevated triglycerides by 15%. Every 30 minutes of lifestyle activity reduced the risk by 15%.
⇀ Consider the reflexology solution
  · Foot reflexology resulted in a significant decrease in triglycerides among hypertensive individuals when applied twice a week for six weeks followed by self foot reflexology applied twice a week for four weeks. A strong effect for

high-cholesterol patients was found with application of
reflexology for 30–40 minutes five or six times a week.
➥Consider the tai chi solution
  • A six-month program of kung fu or tai chi resulted in
    reductions in triglycerides for overweight adolescents.
➥Consider the yoga solution
  • Studies show yoga practice amounts of time varying from
    six weeks to 12 months was associated with a 22.0% to
    28.5% reduction in triglycerides.
  • Study participants who practiced one hour of yoga weekly
    for three months showed lower triglyceride levels.

Waistline

Elevated waist circumference is an indicator for cardiovascular
disease, stroke, heart attack, cognitive decline, Alzheimer's
disease, cancer, obesity, and metabolic syndrome.

Reflex activities that increase risk for elevated waistline circumference
➥Sitting time
  • Men who sit more than four hours per day have 88% higher
    odds of elevated waist circumference.
  • More sitting time is significantly associated with greater
    waistline circumference.

Reflex techniques that decrease risk for elevated waistline circumference
➥Take 10,000 steps a day
  • Walking 10,000 steps a day over eight months can decrease
    waistline circumference by two inches.
➥Consider light-intensity physical activity
  • Every 1,000 steps taken during light-intensity physical
    activity reduced the risk of elevated waist circumference by
    16%. Every 30 minutes reduced the risk by 14%.
➥Take breaks in sitting
  • Those who take the most breaks in sitting have smaller
    waistlines by an average of 1.6 inches.
  • Taking breaks has more impact on waistline size than exercise.

Lifestyle conditions

Sitting time is associated with increased risk for lifestyle conditions. Un-sitting provides a blueprint to lessen risk. The basic "dose" helps lessen metabolic and other indicators that put one at risk for multiple lifestyle conditions. Particular lifestyle conditions are of heightened interest for some of us. Increased risk can be created by heredity, life circumstances, and other factors.

Cognitive abilities, dementia, Alzheimer's

Can we build better brains, improving cognitive abilities, as well as lessening cognitive decline and risks for dementia and Alzheimer's? Can we improve creativity and performance? According to researchers, the answer to these questions is, yes.

Being active throughout life is necessary for sharper cognitive abilities and to lessen the risk of dementia and Alzheimer's. Cognitive processes are tied to moving, so un-sitting your life lessens inactivity, improves metabolism, enhances circulation, and improves your walking abilities. All are building blocks for the cognitive abilities.

Paying attention to the lifestyle choices about moving and sitting is especially important for those with a hereditary link to Alzheimer's. Heredity is 46% of the risk for Alzheimer's. Important to all are physical inactivity and choices related to physical activity, which are 38% of the risk for Alzheimer's.

Metabolism is related to increased risk of Alzheimer's, dementia, and cognitive decline including elevated levels of: blood pressure, blood sugar, fats (cholesterol, triglycerides), and lipoprotein lipase (released by postural muscles as we move).

Those with diabetes are twice as likely to develop dementia. Those with elevated blood-sugar levels, but not diabetes, are at increased risk for dementia with the risk rising with the blood-sugar level. Those who are overweight at the age of 50 show a faster cognitive decline over a ten-year period than individuals with normal weight.

Those who are overweight at the age of 50 with two metabolic abnormalities (high blood pressure, cholesterol, blood sugar, or triglycerides) have the cognitive levels of a normal-weight individual with no metabolic abnormalities seven years older.

Reflex activities that increase risk for cognitive decline
→ Sitting time
  • Walking abilities, potentially hampered by an unstable base created over years of sitting, are associated with cognitive abilities. Frequent falls are an early sign of Alzheimer's in the elderly.
  • Slowed walking speed and irregular steps are tied to cognitive decline and signs of increasing dementia.
→ Physical inactivity
  • Risk for Alzheimer's increased by 250% among those who were physically inactive and whose primary recreational activity from ages 40 to 59 was television-watching.
  • Each one hour of television-viewing from the ages 40 to 59 increases the risk of Alzheimer's disease by 1.3 times.
  • Among the elderly, those who are the least physically active in daily activities are 2.3 times more likely to develop Alzheimer's.

Reflex techniques that potentially decrease risk for cognitive decline
→ Take breaks from sitting
  • Take a break from sitting every 20 minutes. Even a minute of standing will help supply more blood to your brain as blood is pushed out of your legs. Also a two-minute break every 20 minutes is associated with improved glucose/blood-sugar levels. Also effective for normalizing blood-sugar levels is taking a 15-minute walking break after each meal. Reminder: the brain utilizes 60% of the resting body's glucose.
  • The potential for falls later in life is lessened by taking a

two-minute break from sitting every 20 minutes to relieve the stress on the musculoskeletal system and prevent the development of an unstable base for walking.

⟼ Consider the rocking-chair solution

- Rocking for 15 minutes twice a day improves balance, walking speed, and rising out of a chair more easily. Try it for six weeks to see significant improvements.
- Rocking-chair use increases circulation of the blood, in particular to the brain, but also to the heart, which impacts blood pressure.

⟼ Move more, build a better brain

- Walk three times a week for 30 to 45 minutes. Over a year you'll see a 2% growth in the part of the brain responsible for memory.
- Exercise twice a week and eat a healthy diet during middle age to reduce by 50% the risk of Alzheimer's in old age.
- Moderate exercise (brisk walking, aerobics, yoga, strength training, or swimming) is linked with a reduction in cognitive impairment. A 39% reduction was seen in those who exercise in their 40s and a 32% reduction for later in life.
- Active older adults (average age 75) were less likely to develop Alzheimer's and "91% less likely to experience declines in memory, concentration and language abilities after five years".

⟼ Consider the cobblestone mat-walking solution

- Significant improvements in ability to control falling as well as better scores on instrumental activities of daily living such as walking, getting up from, and sitting down in, a chair, bathing, dressing, reaching, and carrying items resulted from walking barefoot on a cobblestoned surface for 45 minutes, three times a week, for four months.

⟼ Consider the tai chi solution

- Notable improvements in balance as well as greater reductions in fear of falling were experienced by senior citizens who practiced qigong and tai chi three times a week for six months.

Cancer preventive

Can some cases of cancer be prevented by paying attention to physical inactivity and prolonged periods of sitting? Researchers say yes.

Physical inactivity and prolonged periods of sitting are linked to 21% of breast cancers, 30% of colon cancers, 54% of lung cancers, and 66% of uterine cancers, according to researchers. It is implicated for increased risk of endometrial, ovarian, and prostate cancer as well as increased cancer mortality in women.

Factors thought to link prolonged sitting and cancer risk: metabolic dysfunction (waist circumference, insulin resistance/ elevated glucose), leptin dysfunction, C-reactive protein, obesity, body mass index.

Reflex activities that increase risk for cancer

⇀ Sitting time
- Those "who spent ten or more years in sedentary jobs had twice the risk of colon cancer and a 44% increased risk of rectal cancer, compared with those who never held a sedentary job".
- There is an increased risk of ovarian cancer for women who sat the most at work and while watching television.
- Women who spent seven hours or more per day sitting had an increased risk of endometrial cancer compared to those who sat less than three hours per day.
- For women who sat six or more hours a day during non-work time there was a 30% higher risk of early death by cancer.
- Odds for death by cancer increased by 17% for women who sat more than 11 hours per day compared to those who sat for four hours.

⇀ Television-watching time
- Each hour per day of television-viewing increases risk of death by cancer 9%.

Reflex techniques that decrease risks for cancer

➼ Take breaks in sitting
- Taking breaks in sitting for between one and two minutes lowers "indicators of cancer risk common to many physical activity cancer studies" including waist circumference, insulin resistance, and inflammation.

➼ Light-intensity physical activity
- Light-intensity physical activity (activities of daily living: cooking, washing dishes, ironing, and other routine domestic or occupational tasks done while standing or walking) has a protective effect and is significantly associated with a reduced risk of breast cancer.

➼ Consider the forest-bathing solution
- A three-day, two-night visit to a forest area is described as a "cancer preventive" by researchers, who found it improved natural killer-cell levels in the immune system. The effects lasted 30 days.

Cardiovascular disease, stroke, heart attack

Prolonged periods of sitting are linked to worse metabolic indicators of cardiac function: triglycerides, cholesterol, glucose levels, blood pressure, leptin levels, waist circumference, insulin resistance, abnormal levels of LPL (lipoprotein lipase), and C-reactive protein.

Cardiovascular disease is the leading cause of death in the world, killing more than all other forms of cancer, combined in the US with an estimated cost of $444 billion in 2010. Stroke is the second-leading cause of death in the world and the third-leading cause of death in the US. Concern is raised over an increase in rates of conditions tied to risk for stroke: diabetes, heart disease, and obesity. Cost to treat stroke is estimated to cumulatively total $2.2 trillion over the 45 years ending in 2050 if no action is taken to improve preventive care.

Reflex activities that increase the risk for cardiovascular disease, stroke, and heart attack

➼ Screen time

- An evening of screen time, four hours or more, over four years resulted in a 113% increased risk of heart attack or stroke for men. Men who spent two hours a day in such leisure-time activities were 50% more likely to die of any cause.
➥ Sitting time
  - More sitting time is significantly associated with higher levels of C-reactive protein, for women.
  - "The more people sat, for any reason, the more likely they were to die of heart disease within 12 years – even if they were slim and exercised regularly. [Prolonged sitting] was associated with increased risk of all causes and cardiovascular disease mortality."
  - Odds for death by cardiovascular disorder increased by 15% and death by coronary heart disease by 27% for women who sat more than 11 hours per day compared to those who sat for four hours.
  - Women who sat for more than six hours a day compared with women who sat for fewer than three hours a day had a 33% higher risk of early death from cardiovascular disease. Men who sat for more than six hours a day compared with men who sat for fewer than three hours a day had an 18% increased risk of premature death from heart disease.
➥ Television-watching time
  - Each two hours of television-watching per day results in a 15% increase in risk for fatal or nonfatal cardiovascular disease (stroke, heart attack, or other).
  - Each hour of television-viewing increases by 18% the risk of dying from cardiovascular disease. Watching for four or more hours per day compared to less than one hour a day resulted in an 80% increased risk of dying from cardiovascular disease.

Reflex techniques that decrease risk for cardiovascular disease, stroke, and heart attack

➥ Lessen uninterrupted sitting time
  - It is estimated that reductions in sitting time of between one and two hours a day "could have a substantial (population-wide) impact on the prevention of cardiovascular disease".

➥ Lessen seated and uninterrupted television-watching time
  • One less hour of seated television-watching per day could result in a risk reduction for coronary heart disease of 2.5% and stroke of 4%. Watching less than two hours per day plus exercising one hour per week could result in a 12.6% reduction in the risk of coronary heart disease and a 20.4% reduction in stroke risk.
➥ Take breaks in sitting
  • Even one minute of standing made a difference in "various indicators of risk for heart disease, metabolic diseases such as diabetes, and inflammatory processes that can play a role in atherosclerosis (blocked arteries)".
  • "Individuals who took the most breaks in sitting showed smaller waistlines (1½ inches) and reduced levels of C-reactive protein, a marker for heart disease indicating inflammation."
  • Higher glucose levels after eating are a risk factor for cardio-vascular disease. Research shows taking breaks in sitting of

LOWER LONG-TERM DIASTOLIC BLOOD PRESSURE

Prolonged differences in one's long-term average diastolic blood pressure is associated with less stroke and coronary heart disease. Multiple reflex techniques contribute to lessening blood pressure and cardiovascular risk. See Chapter Four for reflex activities that lower blood pressure and reduce risk for cardiovascular disease.

A five-point reduction is associated with 34% less stroke; a 7.5-point reduction is associated with 46% less stroke; 10 points is associated with 56% less stroke.

A five-point reduction is associated with 21% less coronary heart disease; a 7.5 point reduction is associated with 29% less coronary heart disease; a ten-point reduction is associated with 37% less coronary heart disease.

two minutes every 20 minutes helps blood sugar stay level after eating.
  • Taking breaks in sitting helps provide more blood to the heart, lessening risk for high blood pressure.
⇒ Take steps
  • Men who walked 10,000 steps or more a day for eight months decreased their odds of cardiovascular disease by 69%.
  • Walking 10,000 steps a day for 12 weeks lowered the diastolic blood pressure by eight points.
⇒ Consider the electric foot-vibrating platform, foot-roller, and foot-bath solutions
  • Use of an electric foot-vibrating platform, an electric foot roller or a foot bath significantly improves heart-rate variability, the interval between heart beats. Decreased heart-rate variability is associated with a sedentary lifestyle as well as increased risk of cardiovascular disease.
⇒ Consider the forest-bathing solution
  • A two-hour walk in a forest or a densely planted city park significantly reduced several indicators associated with reduced risk of heart attack, including blood pressure, compared to walking in an urban setting.
  • A two-hour walk in the forest significantly increased several indicators associated with reduced risk of heart attack (blood pressure and the hormone adiponectin) as compared to a two-hour walk in a city.
  • Forest-bathing, a seven-day trip to a forest resulted in benefits therapeutic for elderly hypertensive patients compared to a seven-day period in a city environment. Tested were blood pressure, cardiovascular disease-related factors as well as C-reactive protein.
⇒ Consider the tai chi solution
  • A six-month program of kung fu or tai chi training "increased lean body mass was related to reductions in insulin resistance, triglycerides, and total cholesterol" as well as decreased C-reactive protein for overweight adolescents.

Depression

Reflex activities that increase risk of depression

➥ Sitting time

- One writer notes the result of sitting too much: "You're also more prone to depression: With less blood flow, fewer feel-good hormones are circulating to your brain."
- Depression was experienced the most by those who sat the most and engaged in moderate to vigorous physical activity the least. Especially impacted were overweight and obese adults.

Reflex techniques that decrease risk for depression

➥ Consider the reflexology solution

- Multiple studies show an improvement in mood or lessening of depression with the application of reflexology.

➥ Consider the forest-bathing solution

- Taking a walk in the forest significantly decreased anxiety, depression, and anger. A two-hour walk in a city park with a good density of trees can produce this effect.

➥ Consider the tai chi solution

- One hour of tai chi three times per week for 12 weeks was associated with "significant improvements in ... depressive symptoms, and... general health, mental health and vitality subscores."

➥ Take 10,000 steps a day

- Of individuals who increased their number of steps to 10,000 a day, 35% indicated they had gained confidence in themselves, which researchers infer reduces the likelihood of depression and anxiety.

Diabetes prevention/glucose/blood sugar/ glucose tolerance/insulin sensitivity/insulin resistance

See pages 132–6.

Erectile dysfunction/infertility/reproductive concerns

Reproductive concerns are linked to a sedentary lifestyle.

Reflex activities that increase the problem
➥ Television-watching time
- A 44% lower sperm count was found for male college students among those who watched more than three hours of television per day.

➥ Sitting time
- More than half of taxi drivers in Beijing suffer from erectile dysfunction, a new government survey has indicated. "In total, 350 men were questioned by the China Family Planning Association, the *Wall Street Journal* reports. The CHPA believes that prolonged sitting may be causing the problem."
- Sperm count is reduced for men who sit for over two hours at a time when working.
- Chinese researchers cite lack of circulation and, for women, lack of ventilation, when relating prolonged sitting to a variety of disorders of the reproductive organs: infertility, cervititis, cervical erosion, sub-cervical hypertrophy, cervical polyps, pre-menstrual and menstrual-period severe pain, dysmenorrhea, fallopian tube obstruction, endometriosis, prostatitis, and vaginitis.

Longevity
Want to live longer? Sit less. Some 27% of deaths from all causes in the US are associated with sitting too much and 19% of deaths are associated with excessive television-viewing.

Reflex activities that increase risk for a shorter life
➥ Television-viewing time
- One hour of television-viewing shortens life by 22 minutes – the same amount as if one had smoked two cigarettes. Over a lifetime, each hour of television-viewing reduces one's life by 1.8 years for men and 1.5 years for women. Those who watch an average of six hours a day over a lifetime can expect to live 4.8 years less. At the most extreme, those who watch the most television reduce their lives by 44 minutes for each hour of viewing for a total of up to 10.4 years, in comparison to those who watch no television.

- Watching television for more than four hours per day resulted in an 80% increased risk of dying from cardiovascular disease compared to those who watched for less than one hour a day.
- Those who watch television for more than four hours a day were 46% more likely to die of any cause, compared to people who watch for less than two hours a day.
- "The more people sat, for any reason, the more likely they were to die of heart disease within 12 years – even if they were slim and exercised regularly."
- For every two hours of television-viewing, a 13% increase in risk of early death resulted.

⇥ Screen time
- A 50% increased risk of premature death was found in men who spent more than four hours a day in non-work-related screen time (TV viewing, surfing the internet or playing video games).

⇥ Sitting time
- Sitting more than six hours a day compared to three hours a day results in: 37% reduction in life expectancy for women and 18% reduction in life expectancy for men.
- Sitting down for more than three hours a day reduces life expectancy by two years.
- There is a consistent link between "chair time" and deaths from heart disease: "The more people sat, for any reason, the more likely they were to die of heart disease within 12 years — even if they were slim and exercised regularly.... all things being equal (body weight, physical activity levels, smoking, alcohol intake, age, and sex) the person who sits more is at a higher risk of death (by any cause) than the person who sits less," according to researchers.

Metabolic syndrome

Metabolic syndrome is a group of factors which serve as indicators of risk for cardiovascular disease and other health problems. People with metabolic syndrome are two to three times as likely to develop heart disease and type-two diabetes; twice as likely to suffer a heart attack or stroke; and more than three times as likely to die early from those causes. Those with multiple metabolic risk factors in middle age have poorer cognitive function, suggestive of dementia or Alzheimer's, later in life.

Approximately 33% of middle-aged people in the Western world experience metabolic syndrome. In America, 25% of all Americans, 12% of children, and 50% of those over the age of 60 experience metabolic syndrome. Researchers see obesity and inactivity as being responsible for a rise in the syndrome.

The metabolic biomarkers are triglycerides, HDL (good) cholesterol, glucose (blood sugar), blood pressure, and waist size. These biomarkers are associated with energy expenditure and how we process sugars and fats. Individuals with abnormal measurements for three of the five biomarkers, such as high blood pressure, large waistline, and poor cholesterol, have metabolic syndrome.

For more information about individual metabolic biomarkers, see Biomarkers at the beginning of this chapter.

Reflex activities that increase risk for metabolic syndrome
➥ Sitting time
  · The more the sedentary behavior, the worse the indicators of metabolic syndrome. Reducing uninterrupted sitting time to less than one hour a day would reduce metabolic syndrome among American adults by 30–35%.
➥ Television-viewing time
  · Each hour of television-viewing increases the risk of metabolic syndrome by 21% for women and 26% for men.
➥ Screen time
The risks for having metabolic syndrome increased for men with more screen time.
  · One hour per day: 41% greater risk
  · Two hours per day: 37% greater risk
  · Three hours per day: 70% greater risk
  · Four hours per day: double the risk for men who do not exercise.

Men with more than four hours per day screen time outside of work have:
- 94% higher odds (virtually double) of having metabolic syndrome.
- 88% higher odds of elevated waist circumference.
- 84% higher odds of low high-density lipoprotein cholesterol (HDL-C).
- 55% higher odds of high blood pressure.
- 32% higher odds of elevated glucose (two to three hours/day).

- Women with more than four hours per day screen time outside of work who do not exercise 30 minutes a day have 54% higher odds of metabolic syndrome. This risk is smaller than that for men. The researcher hypothesized that women take more breaks from sitting.

Reflex techniques that decrease risk for metabolic syndrome

➥ Take breaks in sitting
- Taking breaks in sitting re-sets metabolic mechanisms of the body, improving cholesterol, triglycerides, waistline, insulin resistance, and glucose. In general, those who take the most breaks during the day, even for one minute, had better biomarkers for metabolism and a lessened risk for heart disease and diabetes.
- It is better to take a break in sitting of two minutes, with movement or walking in place, every 20 minutes. Even 30 seconds of standing will impact blood-sugar levels.

➥ Take steps
- The odds of having metabolic syndrome are lowered by 13% for every 1,000 steps taken or 30 minutes spent during activities of daily living (cooking, ironing, cleaning, and other routine tasks done while standing or walking).
- Taking 10,000 steps a day can, over eight months, decrease waistline circumference by two inches, result in weight loss of 10 pounds, and reduce high blood pressure by 34%.
- Those taking 1,350 steps compared to 10,000 steps a day showed worse metabolizing of fats and sugars and

expanding waist circumferences within two weeks.
➥ Consider the tai chi solution
  • One hour of tai chi three times per week for 12 weeks was
    associated with significant improvements in indicators of
    metabolic syndrome including waist circumference, blood
    pressure, and insulin resistance.

Musculoskeletal discomfort/pain/mobility/falls

Reflex activities that increase risk for musculoskeletal stress
➥ Sitting time
  • Sitting too much impacts muscles, tendons, and ligaments
    creating musculoskeletal discomfort and pain and over a
    lifetime impacting fluid gait and maintaining the lower back
    as a stable base for walking.
  • Hip flexors hold the pelvis and lower back in place, helping
    to create a stable base for standing and walking. Sitting too
    much tightens these muscles. Some consider tightened hip
    flexors to be the cause of back pain for many. Over time,
    the lower back becomes a less stable base for standing or
    walking, impacting mobility and risk for falls.

Reflex techniques that decrease risk for musculoskeletal stress
➥ Take breaks in sitting
  • Taking two-minute breaks every 20 minutes relieves the
    stress of sitting for the musculoskeletal system – lessening
    tension in major muscle groups and joints, decompressing
    pressure on the spine, and helping prevent deformation of
    ligaments.
  • Micro-breaks of 30 seconds, taken at 20-minute intervals
    during computer work, had a positive effect on reducing
    discomfort in neck muscles, lower-back muscles, trapezius
    muscles, wrist, and fingers, with no detriment to productivity.
  • Also effective at relieving musculoskeletal discomfort
    are: a five-minute break every hour (aside from mid-
    morning, mid-afternoon, and lunch breaks); four breaks an
    hour; 30-second micro-breaks and a three-minute break.
    Stretching and/or walking away from the work station are
    suggested.

⟿ Consider the rocking-chair solution
  • A six-week program of rocking twice a day for 15 minutes created significant improvements in movement-related activities such as balance, walking speed, and rising out of a chair for elderly women.
  • Less pain medication was requested by the elderly who rocked an accumulated time of 70 minutes during the day.
⟿ Consider the reflexology solution
  • Pain reduction is a significant result of reflexology work. Twenty-seven studies show positive outcomes for reflexology work, ranging from "significant difference in" pain to "reduction in" pain.
⟿ Consider the cobblestone-mat solution
  • Pain was reduced for senior citizens who walked on cobblestone reflexology mats three times a week for 45 minutes over four months.
⟿ Consider the tai chi solution
  • Arthritis patients who practiced tai chi twice a week for 12 weeks experienced less pain during the activities of daily living.
  • Separate research studies have found a reduction in falls, fear of falling, and risk of falls among those who practice tai chi. Twelve weeks of tai chi practice improved the arthritic symptoms, balance, and physical functioning in older women with osteoarthritis.

Osteoporosis

Research has not shown how much sitting and un-sitting lessen the risk of osteoporosis. As a general rule, the more one is up and about, standing and moving around, the more demand is put on bones, thus lessening the risk of osteoporosis.

Weight

When we're up and about as much as intended by our body's evolutionary design, the mechanisms that manage our weight for us are able to go about their work. Un-sitting your life – two hours more a day up and about, with two-minute breaks every 20 minutes – not only helps you expend more calories but also builds toward re-setting metabolic mechanisms thrown off by prolonged sitting.

As you make decisions about moving more throughout your day, be mindful of what you are gaining. By consciously considering what you spend your time doing, you are gaining control of what you may have considered an out-of-control situation, your weight. Every footstep and every break in sitting activates postural muscles and pressure sensors, requesting your body to go to work for you. Information about the impact on weight of reflex activities and reflex techniques is noted below. First we discuss general targets that provide solutions for addressing weight.

Targets for addressing weight

⤳ Target: substitute activity for sitting
  • Move two to two and a half hours more a day than you do currently. This is the equivalent of expending 200 calories a day. Remember, the sedentary office lifestyle is thought to be responsible for 100 less calories expended per day and, when paired with sedentary entertainment in the evening, is ultimately responsible for the culture-wide weight gain.

⤳ Target: expend more calories
  • If you're interested in, and motivated by, the calorie count of un-sitting your life, that information is available. See below.

⤳ Target: re-set metabolism
  • Sitting too much is linked to dis-regulation of the biomarkers for metabolism. Dis-regulation of metabolism contributes to weight gain and obesity. Biomarkers for metabolism include: "good" cholesterol, triglycerides, glucose levels, blood pressure, leptin, and waist circumference.
  • Total sitting time is crucial to metabolizing fats. Taking breaks is important to metabolizing sugars. As you target your sitting time, you are targeting triglyceride and cholesterol levels. As you consider taking breaks, you are targeting glucose levels as well as blood pressure and waistline. Those who take more breaks have smaller waistlines, found to be more important than exercising.

➥ Target: address leptin resistance
- Leptin resistance is associated with obesity, fat regulation, and appetite control. Leptin is a hormone produced by fat cells, released to the bloodstream and circulating to the brain as indicator for the body's appetite control. Leptin resistance occurs "as leptin levels rise in association with increased fat reserves, fail-safe mechanisms built into the body reduce the effectiveness of leptin signaling".
- Total sitting time is related to leptin and leptin resistance.

Reflex activities that increase risk for weight gain
➥ Sitting time at work
- Each two-hour day increment in sitting at work presents 5% increase in risk of obesity.
➥ Television-watching time
- For each hour per day of television-watching there was a one-third pound weight gain for each hour of television-watching at the end of four years for those who watched between four and 11 hours per day. The average weight gain was 3.4 pounds for participants over the four years, which corresponds to a weight gain of nearly 17 pounds over 20 years.
- For each two hours per day of television-viewing there was a 23% increase in the risk of obesity for women.
- For one to two and a half hours' television-viewing compared to less than one hour per day, 93% were more likely to be overweight and 60% had an increased risk of obesity for men.
- For one to three hours per day television-viewing, there was a 42% increased risk of obesity.
- More than two hours per day of television-viewing increases risk of insulin-resistance, obesity, and abnormal concentrations of cholesterol, triglycerides, and other lipids in the blood.
- For two and half to four hours' television-viewing time per day, compared to less than one hour a day, 183% were more likely to be overweight.
- More than three hours a day, among study participants,

those who exercised the least and who watched the most television had a 90% increased risk of obesity.
- Those who exercise and watch more than three hours of television each day are as fat as those who don't exercise.
- Three to four hours a day of television-viewing produce twice the prevalence of obesity.
- More than four hours a day of television-viewing produces more than double the increased risk of obesity for women and four times more likely to be overweight
- Those who exercised and watched four hours of television per day were twice as likely to be overweight compared to those who watched less than one hour of television per day and who did or did not exercise.
- Six or more hours a day of television-viewing produced double the risk of obesity for women and men were four times more likely to be overweight than those who watched an hour or less per week.

Reflex techniques that decrease the risk of weight gain

Following the minimum "dose" will provide your basic "diet". The reflex techniques that follow provide information so you can be mindful of how what you do impacts your weight.

➥ Take breaks in sitting
- Following the "dosing" rule, taking a two-minute standing or walking break every 20 minutes contributes to re-setting metabolism, in particular normalizing blood glucose and blood pressure as well as impacting waistline.
➥ Move more
- Risk of obesity decreases by 9% for each additional two hours per day spent walking or standing at home. Each one-hour per day "increase in brisk walking (moderate physical activity) was associated with a 24% reduction in obesity".
➥ Add 2,000 steps a day to your day
- If you add just 2,000 more steps a day to your regular activities, you'll maintain your weight.
➥ Take 10,000 steps a day
- Research demonstrates that walking 10,000 steps a day can:

decrease waistline circumference by two inches, result in weight loss of 10 pounds, and reduce high blood pressure by 34%. Walking 10,000 steps a day for 12 weeks lowered the diastolic blood pressure by eight points.

⟿ Consider the forest-bathing solution.
- Researchers found significantly higher levels of a hormone that increases fat metabolism results when study participants walked in a forest for two hours in the morning and two hours in the afternoon when compared to city walks of the same duration.

⟿ Consider the rocking-chair solution
- Rocking in a rocking chair expends 150 calories per hour compared to the 77 calories of sitting still.

⟿ Consider the cobblestone-mat-walking solution
- Chinese researchers report results from the use of cobblestone mat-walking (stepping-stone fitness) as a "functional diet" with weight loss taking place as functions of the body improve over time as one walks on a cobblestoned surface. It is seen to produce a "diet effect" as stimulation of the feet improves blood circulation, aids in the metabolism of fats, conditions nerve and endocrine function as well as reducing appetite.
- It is suggested that 30 minutes of stepping-stone fitness per day reduces the appetite by half. Stepping-stone walking is noted as having "been tested by experts, who suggest possible weight loss of 20–30 pounds after a year of 30-minute daily stepping-stone walking".

⟿ Consider the tai chi solution
- A study showed overweight adolescents provided with a six-month program of kung fu or tai chi training "Increased lean body mass was related to reductions in insulin resistance, triglycerides, and total cholesterol".

⟿ Consider the yoga solution
- Studies show yoga practice over amounts of time varying from four weeks to 12 months "was associated with a 1.5% to 13.6% reduction in body weight". It is estimated that people typically gain about one pound per year between the ages of 45 and 55. Individuals who practiced yoga weekly for

four years at least experienced a three-pound reduction in expected weight gain.

➥ Consider using a standing desk at the office

- Standing burns 40% more calories than sitting, which translates to weight loss for a 175-pound person in the following way:
- Standing for two and a half hours each day would result in an extra energy expenditure of 350 calories per day.
- It takes 3,500 calories to equal one pound of weight loss.
- Ten days of 350 calories per day equals one pound of weight loss.
- There are 250 working days in a year or the potential for 20–25 pounds of weight loss by adopting this method of working."

➥ Take breaks in sitting throughout the day

- Taking breaks in sitting expends between 24 and 132 calories during an eight-hour day at the office, depending on how much break you take each hour.
- A one-minute break every half hour results in the expenditure of an additional 24 calories over an eight-hour time period.
- A two-minute break every half hour results in 59 extra calories expended.
- A five-minute break every half hour results in 132 additional calories expended.

➥ Take stepping breaks during commercials in TV-viewing

- An hour of television-viewing can add up to 148 calories expended and 2,000 steps taken when you stand up and walk in place during commercial breaks.
- An hour of television-watching includes 16 to 24 minutes of commercials. Stepping in place during one hour of commercials resulted in an average of about 25 minutes of physical activity. This is 67 more calories than the 81 calories expended while watching television for an hour in a reclined position and 69 more than the 79 calories while watching during an hour of uninterrupted sitting.

SOLUTIONS SUMMARY

Condition	Reflex activities that increase risk	Reflex techniques that decrease risk
Elevated blood pressure	Television-watching time	Take 10,000 steps Take breaks in sitting The cobblestone mat-walking solution The rocking-chair solution The reflexology solution The tai chi solution The yoga solution The massage sandal-wearing solution The forest-bathing solution
Elevated cholesterol	Sitting time	Take lifestyle steps Take breaks in sitting The reflexology solution The yoga solution The tai chi solution
Elevated C-reactive protein	Seated and uninterrupted screen-viewing time Uninterrupted sitting time	Take lifestyle steps Take breaks in sitting The forest-bathing solution The tai chi solution
Elevated glucose levels	Sitting time Walking less than 3,000 steps a day Television-watching time Screen-viewing time	Take breaks in sitting Light-physical-intensity activity, moderate-to-vigorous physical intensity The electric foot vibrator, foot-roller, and foot-bath solution The reflexology solution The tai chi solution The yoga solution
Elevated leptin levels/ leptin resistance	Television-watching time Sitting time	Lessen sitting time
Abnormal lipoprotein lipase levels	Sitting time	Lessen sitting time

SOLUTIONS SUMMARY CONTINUED

Condition	Reflex activities that increase risk	Reflex techniques that decrease risk
Elevated triglyceride levels	Television-watching time	Take breaks in sitting Take steps Consider the reflexology solution Consider the tai chi solution Consider the yoga solution
Elevated waistline circumference	Sitting time	Take 10,000 steps a day Consider light-intensity physical activity Take breaks in sitting
Cognitive decline	Sitting time Television-watching time Physical inactivity	Take breaks from sitting The rocking-chair solution Move more The cobblestone mat-walking solution The tai chi solution
Cancer	Sitting time Television-watching time	Take breaks in sitting Light-intensity physical activity The forest-bathing solution
Cardiovascular disease, stroke, heart attack	Screen time Sitting time Television-watching time	Lessen uninterrupted sitting time Lessen seated and uninterrupted television-watching time Take breaks in sitting Take steps The electric foot-vibrating platform, foot-roller, and foot-bath solutions The forest-bathing solution The tai chi solution
Depression	Sitting time	The reflexology solution The forest-bathing solution The tai chi solution Take 10,000 steps a day

SOLUTIONS SUMMARY CONTINUED

Condition	Reflex activities that increase risk	Reflex techniques that decrease risk
Erectile dysfunction/ infertility/reproductive concerns	Television-watching Sitting time	
Longevity	Television-watching Screen time	
Metabolic syndrome	Sitting time Television-viewing Screen time	Take breaks in sitting Take steps The tai chi solution
Musculoskeletal stress	Sitting time	Take breaks in sitting The rocking-chair solution The reflexology solution The cobblestone mat-walking solution The tai chi solution
Weight gain	Sitting time at work Television-watching	Take breaks in sitting Move more Add 2,000 steps a day to your day Take 10,000 steps a day The forest-bathing solution The rocking-chair solution The cobblestone mat-walking solution The tai chi solution The yoga solution Use a standing desk at the office Take breaks in sitting throughout the day Take stepping breaks during commercial breaks in television-viewing

References

Alzheimer's Association, "New Research Indicates Gait Changes Could Signal Increased Risk For Cognitive Impairment," July 15, 2012

Arney, Katharine, "TV watching 'makes you obese'," BBC News, April 22, 2003, http://news.bbc.co.uk/2/hi/health/2966843.stm

Aronne, Louis J MD, "Role of Leptin in Obesity," January 27, 2011, http:// www.amylin.com/news/online-summit/obesity-perspective/role-of-leptin-in-obesity.htm

Bankhead, Charles, "Trading Stairs for Elevator Seen as Risky to Health," MedPage Today, March 20, 2008

Bartram, Max, "Beijing cabbies suffer erectile dysfunction in silence," April 19, 2011, http://www.121doc.co.uk/news/beijing-cabbies-erectile-dysfunction-5351.html

Benden, Mark E, Blake, Jamilia J, Wendel, Monica L, Huber Jr, John C, "The Impact of Stand-Biased Desks in Classrooms on Calorie Expenditure in Children," *American Journal of Public Health*: August 2011, Vol. 101, No. 8, pp. 1433-1436. doi: 10.2105/AJPH.2010.300072

Bertrais S, Beyeme-Ondoua JP, Czernichow S, Galan P, Hercberg S, Oppert JM "Sedentary behaviors, physical activity, and metabolic syndrome in middle-aged French subjects," 108. Obesity Research 2005, 13:936-44

Blass, Eileen, "More than 90,000 new cancer cases a year in the United States may be due to physical inactivity and prolonged periods of sitting, a new analysis shows."

Boseley, Sarah, "Sedentary lifestyle can lead to pulmonary embolism, study finds," *The Guardian*, July 5, 2011

Bumgardner, Wendy, "Walk 2000 More Steps a Day and Never Gain Another Pound," March 24, 2011, http://walking.about.com/cs/pedometers/a/2000steps.htm

Camhi SM, Sisson SB, Johnson WD, Katzmarzyk PT, Tudor-Locke C, "Accelerometerdetermined lifestyle activity, cardiovascular disease risk factors and metabolic syndrome," (Abstract) Med Sci Sports Exerc 2010;(5 Suppl.):S56

Chang1, Pei-Chia, Tsai-Chung Li2,3,4,5 , Ming-Tsang Wu6, Chiu-Shong Liu7,8, Chia-Ing Li2 , Ching-Chu Chen7,8 , Wen-Yuan Lin7,8 , Shin-Yuh Yang3, and Cheng-Chieh Lin2,5,7,8,9, "Association between television viewing and the risk of metabolic syndrome in a community-based population," BMC Public Health 2008, 8:193doi: 10.1186/1471-2458-8-193

Ching, Pamela LYH, ScD, RD, Walter C Wilet, MD, Eric B Rimm, ScD, Graham A Colditz, MBBS, Steven L Gotmaker, PhD, and Meir J Stampfer, MD, "Activity Level and Risk of Overweight in Male Health Professionals," *American Journal of Public Health*, January 1996, Vp;. 86, No. 1

Church TS, Thomas DM, Tudor-Locke C, Katzmarzyk PT, Earnest CP, Rodarte RQ, Martin CK, Blair SN, Bouchard C, "Trends over 5 decades in U.S. occupation-related physical activity and their associations with obesity," PLoS One. 2011;6(5):e19657. Epub 2011 May 25

Dreyfuss, Ira, "Exercise Can Reduce Diabetes Risk," June 20, 1999, http://www.commercialalert.org/issues/culture/television/exercise-can-reduce-diabetes risk

Dunstan, DW, Barr EL, Healy GN, Salmon J, Shaw JE, Balkau B, Magliano DJ, Cameron AJ, Zimmet PZ, Owen N, "Television viewing time and mortality: the Australian Diabetes, Obesity and Lifestyle Study (AusDiab)." Circulation 2010;121:384–39

Dunstan DW, Zimmet PZ, Welborn TA, Cameron AJ, Shaw J, de Courten M, Jolley D, McCarty DJ; Australian Diabetes, Obesity and Lifestyle Study (AusDiab), Diabetes Res Clin Pract. 2002 Aug;57(2):119-29

Dunstan DW, Kingwell BA, Larsen R, Healy GN, Cerin E, Hamilton MT, Shaw JE, Bertovic DA, Zimmet PZ, Salmon J, Owen N, "Breaking Up Prolonged Sitting Reduces Postprandial Glucose and Insulin Responses," *Diabetes Care.* 2012 Feb 28

Dunstan DW, Salmon J, Owen N, Armstrong T, Zimmet PZ, Welborn TA, Cameron AJ, Dwyer T, Jolley D, Shaw JE; AusDiab Steering Committee, "Associations of TV viewing and physical activity with the metabolic syndrome in Australian adults," Diabetologia. 2005 Nov;48(11):2254-61. Epub 2005 Oct 7

Ferreri, Deana, "Stand up, walk around, and cut down on inflammation," February 16, 2011, http://www.diseaseproof.com/archives/cat-inflammation.html

Ford, Earl S, Kohl III, Harold W, Mokdad, Ali H, Ajani, Umed A, "Sedentary Behavior, Physical Activity, and the Metabolic Syndrome among U.S. Adults," Obesity Research (2005) 13, 608–614; doi: 10.1038/oby.2005.65

Franco JR, Jacobs K, Inzerillp C, Kluzik J, "The effect of the Nintendo Wii Fit and exercise in improving balance and quality of life in community dwelling elders," Technol Health Care. 2012;20(2):95-115. doi: 10.3233/THC-2011-0661

Fung, Teresa T, Hu, Frank B, Yu, Jie, Chu, Nain-Feng, Spiegelman, Donna, Tofler, Geoffrey H, Willett, Walter C, Rimm, Eric B, "Leisure-Time Physical Activity, Television Watching, and Plasma Biomarkers of Obesity and Cardiovascular Disease Risk," *American Journal of Epidemiology* (2000) 152 (12): 1171-1178 doi:10.1093/aje/152.12.1171

Galinsky TL, Swanson NG, Sauter SL, Hurrell JJ, Schleifer LM, "A field study of supplementary rest breaks for data-entry operators," Ergonomics. 2000 May;43(5): 622-38

Gao, Xiang MD, PHD, Nelson, Miriam E PHD, Tucker, Katherine L, "Television Viewing is Associated With Prevalence of Metabolic Syndrome in Hispanic Elders," doi: 10.2337/dc06-1835, Diabetes Care March 2007 vol. 30 no. 3 694-700

Gardiner, Paul A, Healy, Genevieve N, Eakin, Elizabeth G, Clark, Bronwyn K, Dunstan David W, Shaw, Jonathan E, Zimmet, Paul Z, Owen, Neville, "Associations Between Television Viewing Time and Overall Sitting Time with the Metabolic Syndrome in Older Men and Women: The Australian Diabetes Obesity and Lifestyle Study," *The American Geriatrics Society Journal of the American Geriatrics Society,* Volume 59, Issue 5, pages 788–796, May 2011

Gerr F, Marcus M, Ensor C, Kleinbaum D, Cohen S, Edwards A, Gentry E, Ortiz DJ, Monteilh C, "A prospective study of computer users: I. Study design and incidence of musculoskeletal symptoms and disorders, Am J Ind Med. 2002 Apr;41(4):221-35.

Gortmaker, Steven L PhD, Must, Aviva PhD, Sobol, Arthur M AM, Peterson, Karen RD, ScD, Colditz, Graham A MD, DrPH, Dietz, William H MD, PhD, "Television Viewing as a Cause of Increasing Obesity Among Children in the United States, 1986-1990," Arch Pediatr Adolesc Med. 1996;150(4):356-362

Grøntved, Anders MPH, MSc, Hu, Frank B MD, PhD, "Television Viewing and Risk of Type 2 Diabetes, Cardiovascular Disease, and All-Cause Mortality," JAMA. 2011;305(23):2448-2455. doi:10.1001/jama.2011.812

Gustat J, Srinivasan SR, Elkasabany A, Berenson GS: "Relation of self-rated measures of physical activity to multiple risk factors of insulin resistance syndrome in young adults: the Bogalusa Heart Study," J Clin Epidemiol. 2002 Oct;55(10):997-1006

Healy GN, Dunstan DW, Salmon J, Shaw JE, Zimmet PZ, Owen N, "Television time and continuous metabolic risk in physically active adults," Med Sci Sports Exerc. 2008;40: 639-45

Healy GN, Dunstan DW, Salmon J, et al., "Breaks in sedentary time: Beneficial associations with metabolic risk," Diabetes Care. 2008;31:661–666

Healy GN, Wijndaele K, Dunstan DW, Shaw JE, Salmon J, Zimmet PZ, Owen N, "Objectively measured sedentary time, physical activity, and metabolic risk: the Australian Diabetes, Obesity and Lifestyle Study (AusDiab)," Diabetes Care 2008;31:369–371

Healy GN, Owen, "Sedentary Behaviour and Biomarkers of Cardiometabolic Health Risk in Adolescents: An Emerging Scientific and Public Health Issue," Rev Esp Cardiol.2010; 63 :261-4 - Vol.63 Núm 03 DOI: 10.1016/ S1885-5857(10)70057-8

Healy GN, Dunstan DW, Salmon J, Cerin E, Shaw JE, Zimmet PZ, Owen N, "Objectively measured light-intensity physical activity is independently associated with 2-h plasma glucose," Diabetes Care. 2007 Jun;30(6):1384-9. Epub 2007 May 1

Heffernan, Andrew, "The Perfectly Balanced Body," October 28, 2011, http://www. rodalewellness.com/fitness/perfectly-balanced-body

Hu FB, Li TY, Colditz GA, Willett WC, Manson JE. "Television watching and other sedentary behaviors in relation to risk of obesity and type 2 diabetes mellitus in women" JAMA 2003;289:1785–1791 Abstract

Hu FB, Leitzmann MF, Stampfer MJ, Colditz GA, Willett WC, Rimm EB, "Physical activity and television watching in relation to risk for type 2 diabetes mellitus in men". Arch Intern Med 2001;161:1542–1548 Abstract

Jakes RW, Day NE, Khaw KT, Luben R, Oakes S, Welch A, Bingham S, Wareham NJ. "Television viewing and low participation in vigorous recreation are independently associated with obesity and markers of cardiovascular disease risk: EPIC-Norfolk population-based study," Eur J Clin Nutr 2003;57:1089–1096

James, Julia, "High school students sit for too long, new health research suggests," Peninsula Press (CA), Apr 10, 2011

Judson, Olivia, "Stand Up While You Read This!" February 23, 2010, http:// opinionator. blogs.nytimes.com/2010/02/23/stand-up-while-you-read-this/?hp

Katzmarzyk, Peter T, "Physical Activity, Sedentary Behavior, and Health: Paradigm Paralysis or Paradigm Shift?" Diabetes. 2010 Nov;59(11):2715-6.PMID: 2098047

Katzmarzyk PT, Church TS, Craig CL, Bouchard C, "Sitting time and mortality from all causes, cardiovascular disease, and cancer", Med Sci Sports Exerc 2009;41:998–1005

Lajunen, Hanna-Reetta,1 Anna Keski-Rahkonen,#1,2,3 Lea Pulkkinen,#4 Richard J Rose,#1,5 Aila Rissanen,#2 Jaakko Kaprio, "Are computer and cell phone use associated with body mass index and overweight? A population study among twin adolescents," BMC Public Health. 2007; 7: 24.PMCID: PMC1820777

Levine, James A, Lorraine M Lanningham-Foster, Shelly K McCrady, Alisa C Krizan, Leslie R Olson, Paul H Kane, Michael D Jensen, Matthew M Clark, "Interindividual Variation in Posture Allocation: Possible Role in Human Obesity," Science, January 28, 2005:Vol. 307 no. 5709 pp. 584-586 DOI: 10.1126/

science.1106561

Levine, James A, "Nonexercise activity thermogenesis-liberating the life-force," Journal of Internal Medicine, 2007 Sep;262(3):273-87.

Levine, James A, "Q&A: How to drop pounds with all-day activities, not exercise," USA Today, Jan. 21, 2009

Levine JA, Schleusner SJ, Jensen MD, "Energy expenditure of nonexercise activity," Am J Clin Nutr 2000;72:1451–1454 (Abstract)

Levine JA, Vander Weg, Mark W, Hill, James O, Klesges, Robert C, "Non-exercise activity thermogenesis: the crouching tiger hidden dragon of societal weight gain," Arteriosclerosis, Thrombosis, and Vascular Biology 26: 729-736.

Lindstrom HA, Fritsch T, Petot G, Smyth KA, Chen CH, Debanne SM, Lerner AJ, Friedland, RP, "The Relationships between Television Viewing in Midlife and the Development of Alzheimer's Disease in a Case-Control Study," Brain and Cognition, v58 n2 pages 157-165 Jul 2005

Lynch, Brigid M, "Sedentary Behavior and Cancer: A Systematic Review of the Literature and Proposed Biological Mechanisms," Cancer Epidemiol Biomarkers Prev; 19(11); 2691–709

Lynch BM, Friedenreich CM, Winkler EA, Healy GN, Vallance JK, Eakin EG, Owen N, "Breast cancer risk," Breast Cancer Research and Treatment [2011, 130(1):183-94]

Madhavan G, Stewart JM, McLeod KJ: "Effect of plantar microstimulation on cardiovascular responses to immobility", American Journal of Phys. Med. Rehabilitation, 2005, Vol. 84, No. 5, pp. 338-345

Madhavan G, et al., "Cardiovascular systemic regulation by plantar surface stimulation," Biomed Instrum Technol. 2006 Jan-Feb; 40(1):78-84

Manson, JoAnn E, et al., "Walking Compared with Vigorous Exercise for the Prevention of Cardiovascular Events in Women," N Engl J Med 2002; 347:716-725, September 5, 2002

Marcus, Mary Brophy, "Falls linked to early Alzheimer's disease," USA Today, July 17, 2011

Martinez-Gomez, David, Rey-López, Pablo, Chillón, Palma, Gómez-Martínez, Sonia, Vicente-Rodríguez, Germán, Martín-Matillas, Miguel, Garcia-Fuentes, Miguel, Delgado, Manuel, Moreno, Luis A, Veiga, Oscar L, Eisenmann, Joey C, Marcos, Ascension, and AVENA Study Group BMC Public Health., "Excessive TV viewing and cardiovascular disease risk factors in adolescents. The AVENA cross-sectional study" 2010; 10: 274. Published online 2010 May 25. doi: 10.1186/1471-2458-10-274 PMCID: PMC2892447

Mason, Emma, "Study finds more breaks from sitting are good for waistlines and hearts," Jan 11, 2001, http://www.eurekalert.org/pub_releases/2011-01/esoc-sfm010911.php

Mclean L, Tingley M, Scott RN, Rickards J, "Computer terminal work and the benefit of microbreaks," Appl Ergon. 2001 Jun;32(3): 225-37

Mead JR, Irvine, SA, Ramji, DP, "Lipoprotein lipase: structure, function, regulation, and role in disease," J Mol Med (Berl). 2002 Dec;80(12):753-69. Epub 2002 Oct 24.

Meguro, Kenichi, "Gait Changes Correlate with Dementia Symptoms in an 'Old-Old' Population," http://www.sacbee.com/2012/07/15/4632400/new-research-indicates-gaitchanges. html#storylink=cpy

Mitre N, Foster RC, Lanningham-Foster L, Levine JA, "The energy expenditure of an activity-promoting video game compared to sedentary video games and TV watching," J Pediatr Endocrinol Metab. 2011;24(9- 10): 689-95

Mozaffarian, Dariush MD, Dr PH, Hao, Tao MPH, Rimm, Eric B ScD, Willett, Walter C MD, Dr PH, and Hu, Frank B MD, PhD, "Changes in Diet and Lifestyle and Long-Term Weight Gain in Women and Men," New England Journal of Medicine 2011; 364:2392-2404 June 23, 2011

Nygaard H, Tomten SE, Høstmark AT, "Slow postmeal walking reduces postprandial glycemia in middle-aged women," Appl Physiol Nutr Metab. 2009 Dec;34(6):1087-92

Olsen, Rasmus H MD, Krogh-Madsen, Rikke, MD, Thomsen, Carsten, MD, DMSc, Frank W, PhD, Bente K, MD, DMSc, "Metabolic Responses to Reduced Daily Steps in Healthy Nonexercising Men," JAMA, March 19, 2008–Vol 299, No. 11

Ostrow, Nicole, "Walking, Resistance Training May Improve Memory In Study," Jul 15, 2012, http://www.bloomberg.com/news/2012-07-15/walking-resistance-training-mayimprove- memory-in-study.html

Paddock, Catharine, "Prolonged Television Viewing linked to Higher Risk of Death," medicalnewstoday.com, January 12, 2010

Painter, Kim, "Your Health: Too much sitting puts the body on idle," USA Today, 1/31/2010

Pan, Joan, Mashable, Health & Fitness 19 June 2012, http://www.modernghana.com/lifestyle/3383/16/why-sitting-too-much-is-dangerous.

Patel, Alpa V, Leslie Bernstein, Anusila Deka, Heather Spencer Feigelson, Peter T Campbell, Susan M Gapstur, Graham A Colditz, Michael J Thun, "Leisure Time Spent Sitting in Relation to Total Mortality in a Prospective Cohort of US Adults." Am J Epid Published online July 22, 2010 (DOI: 10.1093/aje/kwq155)

Rabin, Roni Caryn, "The Hazards of the Couch," January 12, 2011, http:// well.blogs.nytimes.com/2011/01/12/the-hazards-of-the-couch/

Reynolds, Grechen, "Don't Just Sit There," New York Times Sunday Review, April 28, 2012

Rettner, Rachael, "Frequently breaking up long bouts of sitting with just a few minutes of light exercise helps to lower one's cancer risk," MyHealthNewsDaily, November 3, 2011

Richards, Erin, "Stand-up desks provide a firm footing for fidgety students. Teachers report improved focus, behavior," Journal Sentinel, September 22, 2008 http://www.jsonline.com/news/education/32501809.html

Rosengarden, Craig, "Golf, Fitness and Work? How's your golf game? More importantly, how is your health?" http://online.wsj.com/article/SB118039073511916428.html

Rosenwald, Michael S, "Desk jockeys stand up for standing at work," The Washington Post, October 18, 2010

Saeki Y, Nagai N, Hishinuma M, "Effects of footbathing on autonomic nerve and immune function," Complement Ther Clin Pract. 2007 Aug;13(3):158-65

Salmon J, Bauman A, Crawford D, Timperio A, Owen N, "The association between television viewing and overweight among Australian adults participating in varying levels of leisure-time physical activity," Int J Obes Relat Metab Disord 2000;24:600–606

Shea, Christopher, "Mindful Exercise," The New York Times, December 9, 2007

Sisson SB, Broyles ST, Baker BL, Katzmarzyk PT, "Television, reading, and computer time: correlates of school-day leisure-time sedentary behavior and relationship with overweight in children in the US," J Phys Act Health. 2011 Sep;8 Suppl 2:S188-97

Sisson, Susan B PhD, Camhi, Sarah M PhD, Church, Timothy S MD, MPH, PhD, Martin, Corby K PhD, Tudor-Locke, Catrine PhD,

Bouchard, Claude PhD. Earnest, Conrad P PhD, Smith, Steven R MD, Newton, Jr, Robert L MD, Rankinen, Tuomo PhD, and Katzmarzyk, Peter T PhD, "Leisure Time Sedentary Behavior, Occupational/Domestic Physical Activity, and Metabolic Syndrome in U.S. Men and Women," Metab Syndr Relat Disord. 2009 December; 7(6): 529–536. doi: 10.1089/met.2009.0023 PMCID: PMC2796695 NIHMSID: NIHMS132193

Spalding, Anne, Kelly, Linda, "Rewards for Using Exercise Balls," (Excerpt from Fitness on the Ball), http://www.humankinetics.com/excerpts/excerpts/rewards-forusing-exercise-balls

Stacy, Kelli Miller, "Prolonged Sitting Boosts Bad Health," http://www.webmd.com/fitness-exercise/news/20100119/prolonged-sitting-boosts-bad-health

Stamatakis, Emmanuel Anne PhD, MSc, BSc, Hamer, Mark PhD, MSc, BSc, Dunstan, David W PhD, BAppSc, "Screen-based Entertainment Time, All-cause Mortality, and Cardiovascular Events: Population-based Study With Ongoing Mortality and Hospital Events Follow-up," Journal of the American College of Cardiology. 2011;57(3):292-299

Tokar, Steve, "Over Half of Alzheimer's Cases May Be Preventable, Say Researchers," July 19, 2011, http://www.ucsf.edu/news/2011/07/10278/over-half-alzheimers-may-bepreventable-say-researchers

Tremblay, Mark S1*, Allana G LeBlanc1, Michelle E Kho2, Travis J Saunders1, Richard Larouche1, Rachel C Colley1, Gary Goldfield1, Sarah Connor Gorber3, "Systematic review of sedentary behaviour and health indicators in school-aged children and youth," International Journal of Behavioral Nutrition and Physical Activity 2011, 8:98 doi:10.1186/1479-5868-8-98

Tucker LA, Bagwell M, "Television viewing and obesity in adult females", Am J Public Health 1991;81:908–911

Tucker LA, Friedman GM, "Television viewing and obesity in adult males." Am J Public Health 1989;79:516–518 Abstract/

Vallance, Jeff K, Winkler, Elisabeth A H, Gardiner, Paul A, Healy, Genevieve N, Lynch, Brigid M, Owen, Neville, "Associations of objectively-assessed physical activity and sedentary time with depression: NHANES (2005-2006)," Prev Med. 2011 Oct;53(4-5):284-8

Veerman, J Lennert, Healy, Genevieve N, Cobiac, Linda J, Vos, Theo, Winkler, Elisabeth A H, Owen, Neville, Dunstan, David W, "Television viewing time and reduced life expectancy: a life table analysis," Br J Sports Med doi:10.1136/bjsm.2011.085662

Vlahos, James, "Is Sitting a Lethal Activity?," The New York Times Magazine, April 14, 2011

Wang, Shirley S, "Lifestyle Changes Can Reduce Risk of Alzheimer's," http://online.wsj.com/article/SB10001424052702303795304576454110940969044.html

Warren TY, Barry V, Hooker SP, Sui X, Church TS, Blair SN, "Sedentary behaviors increase risk of cardiovascular disease mortality in men" Med Sci Sports Exerc. 2010 May;42(5):879-85. (Abstract)

Wijndaele K, Brage S, Besson H, et al., "Television viewing time independently predicts all-cause and cardiovascular mortality: the EPIC Norfolk Study", Int J Epidemiol, June 23, 2010

Yates T, Khunti K, Wilmot EG, Brady E, Webb D, Srinivasan B, Henson J, Talbot D, Davies MJ, "Self-reported sitting time and markers of inflammation, insulin resistance, and adiposity," Am J Prev Med. 2012 Jan;42(1):1-7

Links

"TV 'link' to Alzheimer's," Tuesday, March 6, 2001, BBC News Online, http:// news.bbc. co.uk/2/hi/health/1204894.stm

"Prolonged sitting and colon cancer: Study links desk jobs to bowel cancer risk," 20 Apr, 2011, http://www.netdoctor.co.uk/interactive/bth/ article.php?id= %7B8C63ECDA-9938-4A11- B03C- 48A330B4992F%7D&tab_id=224

"Prolonged Sitting Health Risks, Sitting For Long Hours Causes Obesity, Heart Diseases" February 13, 2010, http://www.tandurust.com/ health-research-and-news/healtheffects-of- prolonged-sitting.html

"Physical Activity and Health: A Report of the Surgeon General," http://www.cdc.gov/ nccdphp/sgr/ataglan.htm

Kenkoh (Sandal) Little Earth Study, http:// www.littleearth.co.jp/anti english/kyouto/ index.html

American Institute for Cancer Research, "New Research: Getting Up From Your Desk Can Put the 'Breaks' on Cancer / Experts Urge Americans to Rethink Outdated Notions of Physical Activity, http://www.aicr.org/press/ press-releases/getting-up-from-your-desk.html

"A 10,000 Step Study: 752 participants", http:// chronicdiseaseprevention.org/research/ lancaster/

"Why Exercise Won't Help You Lose Weight," http://www.time.com/time/magazine/ article/0,9171,1914974,00.html

"Study: An hour of TV can shorten your life by 22 minutes," http://www.nbcnews.com/ id/44156412/#.VcPSNkvjPwI

"It's a big day! The world's first evidence- based sedentary behaviour guidelines have been released," February 15, 2011, http:// participaction-en.blogspot.com/2011/02/its- big-dayworlds-first-evidence-based.html

"Breaks in Sedentary Time," http://www. posturepress.com/Posture-Research-6.php

"Long-Term Sedentary Work and the Risk of Subsite-specific Colorectal Cancer," http:// online.wsj.com/article/SB10001424052702303 4992045763878843134027056.html

"Prolonged Televsion Viewing linked to Higher Risk of Death," //www.modernmedicalguide. com/prolonged-tv-viewing-linked-to-higher- risk-of-death/

Acknowledgments

Our thanks to the researchers whose fine work and dedication has brought forward this important field of study. Among those whose work has been particularly helpful are: Dr. Geraldine Healy, Dr. James Levine, Dr. Marc Hamilton, Dr. Peter Katzmarzyk, Dr. Frank B. Hu, Dr.Emmanuel Stamatakis, Dr. Alpa Patel, Dr. Earl Ford, Dr. Mark Benden, Dr. D. W. Dunstan, Dr. Paul A. Gardiner, Dr. Steven Gortmaker, Dr. Guruprasad Madhavan, Dr. Neville Owen, Dr. Susan Sisson, Dr. Sarah M. Camhi, Dr. Mark Tremblay, Dr. Anders Grontved, Dr. Brigid M. Lynch, Dr. Christine M Friedenreich, Dr. RW Jakes, Dr. Carolyn Pierce, Dr Robert Friedland, Dr. Deborah Barnes and Dr. J. Salmon.

Special thanks to Peggy Sadler and Jo Godfrey Wood of Bookworx for their excellent editing and design work.

Made in the USA
Lexington, KY
30 September 2015